Diabetes Care
A Problem Solving Approach

Heather Daly SRN
Diabetes Nurse Specialist, University Hospital, Nottingham

Pat Clarke SRN
Diabetes Nurse Specialist, University Hospital, Nottingham

Joy Field SRN
Ward Sister, University Hospital, Nottingham

Edited by
Tim Dornan MRCP, DM
Senior Registrar, City and University Hospitals, Nottingham

Heinemann Professional Publishing

Heinemann Nursing
An imprint of Heinemann Professional Publishing Ltd
22 Bedford Square, London WC1B 3HH

LONDON MELBOURNE AUCKLAND

First published 1988

British Library Cataloguing in Publication Data
Daly, Heather
Diabetes care.
1. Man. Diabetes – Case studies
I. Title II. Clarke, Pat III. Field,
Joy IV. Dornan, Tim
616.4′62′09

ISBN 0 433 00005 8

Typeset by Eta Services (Typesetters) Ltd, Beccles, Suffolk
and printed in Great Britain by Redwood Burn Ltd, Trowbridge

Preface

Pick up a nursing or medical textbook and it will tell you all about insulin and how it works, but probably nothing about, for example, how to help a child come to terms with having to inject it daily for the rest of his life, and what you do when his frustration and resentment bubbles up to the surface and he truants from school. The gulf between theory and practice creates an aura about diabetes care which threatens to make it an elitist discipline. Yet how can practical knowhow be the preserve of a small elite when up to 2% of the population have the disease and perhaps only a half ever attend hospital clinics? Diabetes concerns all health care workers and more often demands common sense, insight and patience than complex theoretical knowledge. We have distilled from our experience on the wards, in clinics and in the home some of the commoner problems and conjured up fictional people who might experience them. Sometimes we use them to illustrate general points, sometimes we go into more specific problems in detail and offer practical solutions. Background information complementary to the case discussions is highlighted in tinted boxes.

Is this book written on a 'nursing model'? No, nor was it ever intended to be. Diabetes care is the task of a multidisciplinary team where each member knows his/her own and his/her colleagues' roles and limitations. We describe a team approach and illustrate how both specialist and non-specialist nurses can play their part.

We acknowledge with thanks our colleagues who read our first faltering efforts and helped us find our way: Adrian Scott, Simon Heller, Alan Birchall, Ceri Dornan, Jean Bradley, Bernie Kirk, Elisabeth Fletcher, Sally Strang and Julie Noronha. We thank Geoff Lythe, Sally Azadehdel and Wendy Blundell for their help with the illustrations, and Pat Lister who helped to prepare the manuscript with robust good humour. We also thank Eli Lilley for Fig. 1.2. Above all, we thank Robert Tattersall who encouraged us and criticised our efforts from start to finish, and our friends and better halves who put up with us while we were doing the writing.

To Robert Tattersall who got us all interested in diabetes
and taught us much of what we know

(A personal thank you to Tim

with love, Joy, Pat and Heather)

Contents

HOW TO GET THE BEST OUT OF THIS BOOK

The main text in Chapters 3 to 8 is centred around case histories; see the first page of each chapter for a list of them. Practical information is centred in the case discussions; background or theoretical information is given in Chapter 1 or highlighted in boxes like this. For specific points of reference, just use the index.

1/

What is diabetes?

DIABETES MELLITUS: AN HISTORICAL PERSPECTIVE

An illness characterised by raging thirst and excessive urination was described in an Egyptian papyrus as early as 1500 BC. Arataeus, a Greek physician, first used the word 'diabetes' (meaning 'a siphon') nearly 2000 years later to describe the same disease. His phrase 'a melting down of the flesh and limbs into water' describes it accurately; fat and muscle are broken down to glucose which spills from the blood into the urine and 'sucks' water out of the body. Thomas Willis, a 17th-century English physician, noted that the urine was sweet to the taste and added the word 'mellitus' ('honeyed'). In 1889, Von Mering and Minkowski carried out their classical experiment of inducing diabetes in a dog by removing its pancreas, proving that diabetes was linked to the pancreas. At about the same time Langerhans described the small clusters of cells scattered throughout the pancreas that now bear his name (*islets of Langerhans*) and which have since been shown to manufacture insulin (Fig. 1.1). As understanding of the disease increased, so did determination to find a cure. At last in 1922 two young Canadians, Banting (a surgeon) and Best (a medical student), succeeded in isolating and purifying a pancreatic extract which could control diabetes. They called it 'insulin'. This new drug seemed like a miracle; children who would have been condemned to a starvation diet and death within months regained weight, strength and energy and were able to live a normal life (Fig. 1.2).

For the next 10 years only 'soluble' insulin was available. This acted for about 6 h and had to be injected several times a day. Patients still had to stick rigidly to a diet containing little carbohydrate. The 1930s and 1940s saw relaxation of the diet and longer-acting insulin formulations, so that the injections could be given just once a day. In the 1930s, when initial euphoria had

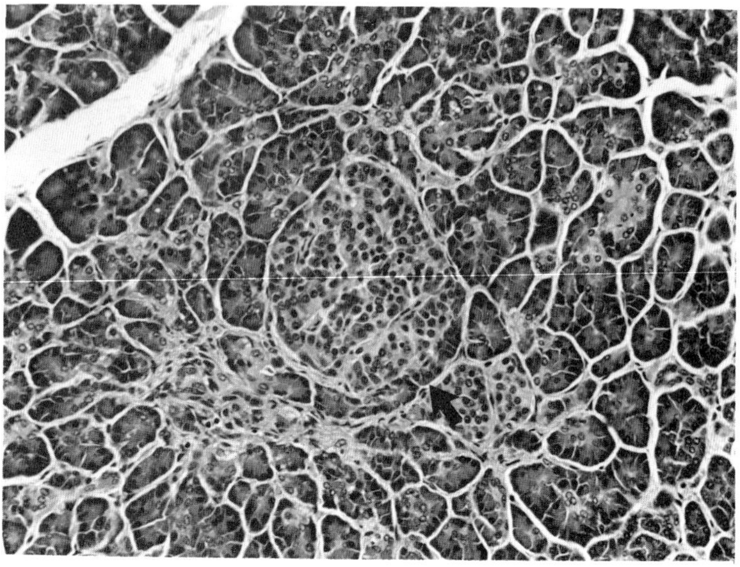

Fig. 1.1 This cross-section of a human pancreas shows an islet of Langerhans (arrowed) surrounded by enzyme-producing tissue.

cooled and insulin was commonplace, a new problem appeared. Patients whose lives had been saved by insulin developed 'late diabetic complications'—blindness, renal failure, heart disease and gangrene. Over 50 years later, we still do not understand what causes these complications and disappointingly little progress has been made in preventing them, although it is generally accepted that the most important measure is to aim for blood glucose levels as close to the non-diabetic state as possible. This is not really very novel because pioneer physicians like Elliott Joslin in the United States and Robin Lawrence in England proposed this half a century ago. Nor are current approaches to insulin treatment very new. Frequent injections of short-acting insulin to imitate the action of the non-diabetic pancreas (see pages 19 and 131) were the norm in the 1920s and have recently come back into vogue.

One other milestone in the history of diabetes was the introduction of oral hypoglycaemic drugs in the late 1950s. Until then, the choice was between diet and insulin; now a treatment other than insulin was available to lower blood glucose and relieve diabetic symptoms in patients with 'maturity-onset diabetes'.

TERMINOLOGY

Arataeus likened his patients to a siphon because they drank so much water (*polydipsia*) and passed so much urine (*polyuria*) that there seemed to be a constant stream of water passing straight through their bodies. Sugar (glucose) in the urine (*glycosuria*) is not the only cause of this siphon. The kidneys regulate output of water from the body under the control of a hormone (*antidiuretic hormone*, or *ADH*) manufactured in the hypothalamus and released into the blood from the pituitary gland. Polyuria and polydipsia can also be caused by shortage of antidiuretic hormone (*cranial diabetes insipidus*) or failure of the kidneys to respond to it (*nephrogenic diabetes insipidus*). In a patient with raging thirst, diabetes insipidus (so called because of the urine's insipid taste!) can easily be distinguished from diabetes mellitus by showing that there is no glucose in the urine. Diabetes insipidus is rare and is not discussed further in this book; the term 'diabetes' is used throughout to mean diabetes mellitus.

WHY DOES DIABETES MATTER?

Ask a man in the street what diabetes means to him and he will probably mention injections, fainting attacks, gangrene or blindness. It is perhaps not surprising that what sticks in his mind is the dramatic side of diabetes. He may be unaware that many patients are treated by diet or tablets alone and that many, including some on insulin, have excellent health and a normal lifespan. His distorted view becomes particularly important if *he* develops diabetes. The first job of his doctor or nurse will be to put a more realistic and encouraging complexion on his illness; however, there is some truth in his view because anyone with diabetes is *at risk* of complications. These include eye disease (*retinopathy*), kidney failure (*nephropathy*), heart attacks, strokes, gangrene (*peripheral vascular disease*) and nerve damage (*neuropathy*), as well as *hyperglycaemiac* (high blood sugar) *coma* and, for women, death of a baby during pregnancy or soon after delivery. Such complications are not inevitable, but the fact that they can occur, even more than the need for lifelong treatment, makes diabetes such an important disease.

It is difficult to give an accurate estimate of the outlook for diabetic patients of the 1980s because current statistics are based on

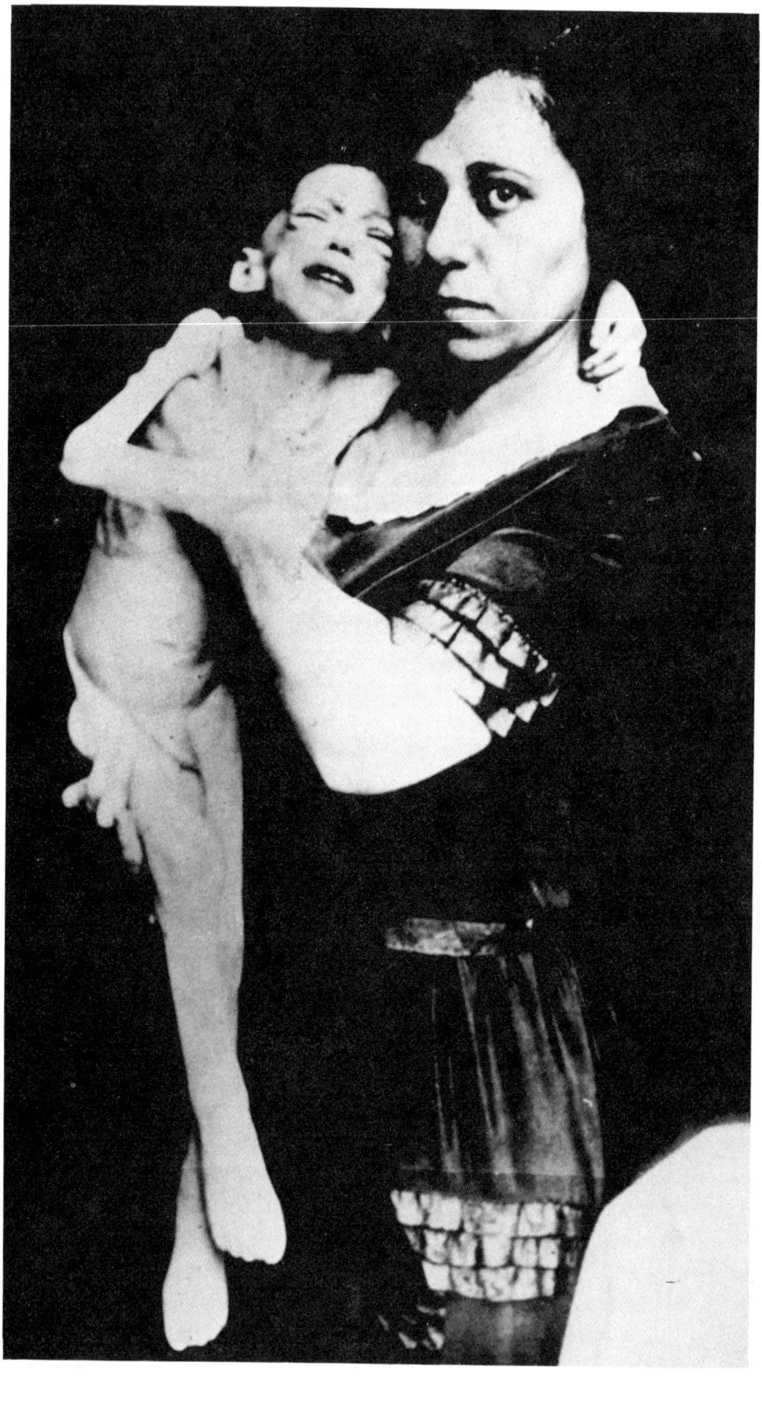

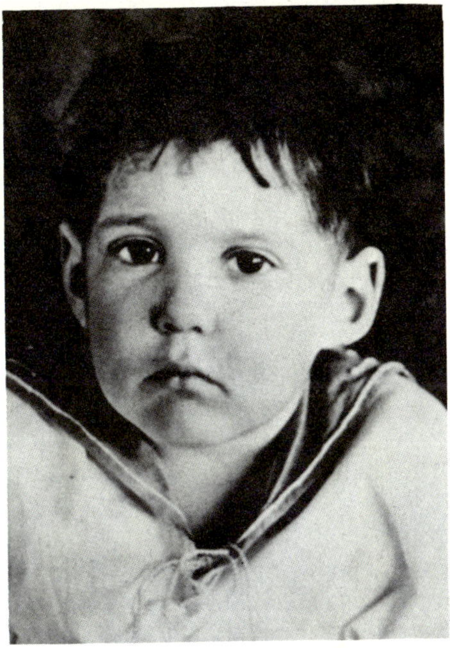

Fig. 1.2 Before and after insulin treatment. Before insulin, JL, age 3 years, weight 6.8 kg, 15 December 1922. After insulin, JL, 15 February 1923, weight 13 kg. These spectacular pictures appeared in the issue of *Journal of the American Medical Association* which introduced insulin to the profession.

people diagnosed many years ago and treatment has changed. In particular, laser treatment for diabetic retinopathy, which can prevent blindness, has only been generally available for 10 years and it is only recently that diabetic patients have been accepted for artificial kidney treatment (renal dialysis and transplants). However, the most recent figures still show diabetes as the commonest cause of blindness in people below the age of 65 and one of the commonest causes of kidney failure. Gangrene and amputations are at least ten times commoner in diabetics than non-diabetics. Heart disease is several times commoner in diabetics than in the general population and is the commonest cause of death. The longer someone has been diabetic, the greater their chance of developing these complications; so those who develop diabetes at the youngest ages have the greatest risk of premature ill-health. People who developed diabetes before 1931 and were aged 30 or less at the time had only a 50% chance of living beyond the age of 55, shortening their life expectancy by nearly 20 years. There is now evidence that eye and kidney disease are becoming less common and it is to be hoped that these trends will continue.

INSULIN: WHAT IS IT AND WHAT DOES IT DO?

Insulin is a hormone produced by only one organ, the pancreas, and by only one type of cell within the pancreas, the beta (or B) cell of the islets of Langerhans (see Fig. 1.1). Insulin is the body's 'storage hormone'. It regulates the laying down of carbohydrate and fat as a reservoir of energy and also helps control the synthesis of protein, the major structural component of the tissues. Diabetes is caused by shortage of insulin, either because the islets simply pack up or because the body demands more insulin than they can supply (see 'Causes and types of diabetes', page 9).

Insulin and carbohydrate metabolism

The two main consumers of energy are muscle and nerves (including the brain and spinal cord); glucose is their principal fuel. Carbohydrate, which constitutes a third to a half the calories in a normal diet, is broken down by enzymes in the gut and absorbed into the blood as glucose. This may be used immediately or, after a large meal, stored in the liver and muscles as *glycogen*, which is readily converted back to glucose and provides an instant energy source. During prolonged fasting, amino acids (the 'building blocks' of which protein is made) and glycerol (the 'skeleton' of molecules of fat) can be converted into glucose by the liver (Fig. 1.3).

The way the pancreas produces insulin to regulate blood glucose in health is like a thermostatically controlled cooling system. As blood glucose rises after a meal, the pancreas switches on insulin production and surplus glucose is stored in muscle and liver as glycogen. During prolonged fasting, blood glucose falls, insulin production shuts down and liver glycogen is broken down to glucose (*glycogenolysis*). A low level of insulin also signals for protein and fat to be broken down and used by the liver to synthesise glucose (*gluconeogenesis*). This system is so efficient that, like the temperature of a fridge, blood glucose varies relatively little in non-diabetic individuals whether they are feasting or fasting.

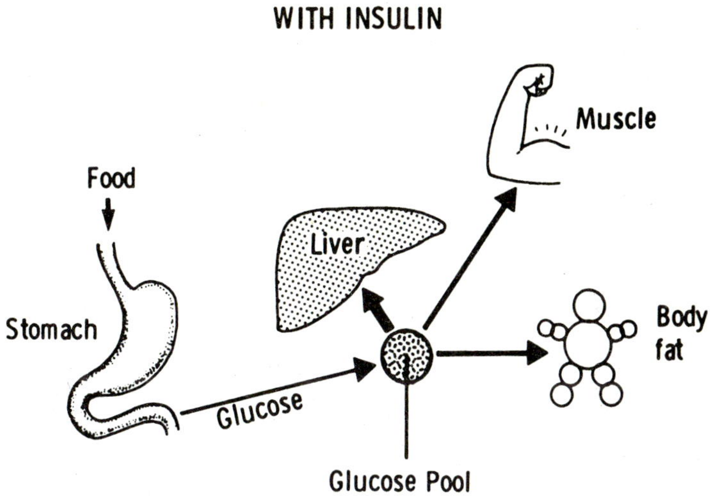

Fig. 1.3 Carbohydrate metabolism in health. When insulin is present, glucose is stored in the liver or fat or burned by the muscles; the glucose pool is small and the level never gets high enough for any to escape into the urine. (Reproduced with permission of Churchill Livingstone.)

Insulin and fat metabolism

Just as insulin lays down surplus carbohydrate in times of plenty, so it encourages fat to be laid down as an energy source. Decreased insulin allows fat to be broken down and used as fuel, both by conversion of glycerol to glucose and by the synthesis of ketones in the liver. Ketones are acidic, so if excessive amounts accumulate in the blood they can make it acid (see page 64).

Insulin and protein metabolism

Production of insulin is a signal that energy is in good supply and protein in the diet can be used to build and repair the tissues. Shortage of insulin redirects dietary protein to the synthesis of glucose (see gluconeogenesis, page 6 above) and also mobilises protein from the tissues.

Insulin deficiency and the symptoms of diabetes

Figure 1.4 shows the effects of insulin deficiency; Table 1.1 shows common symptoms of diabetes. The disease develops when in-

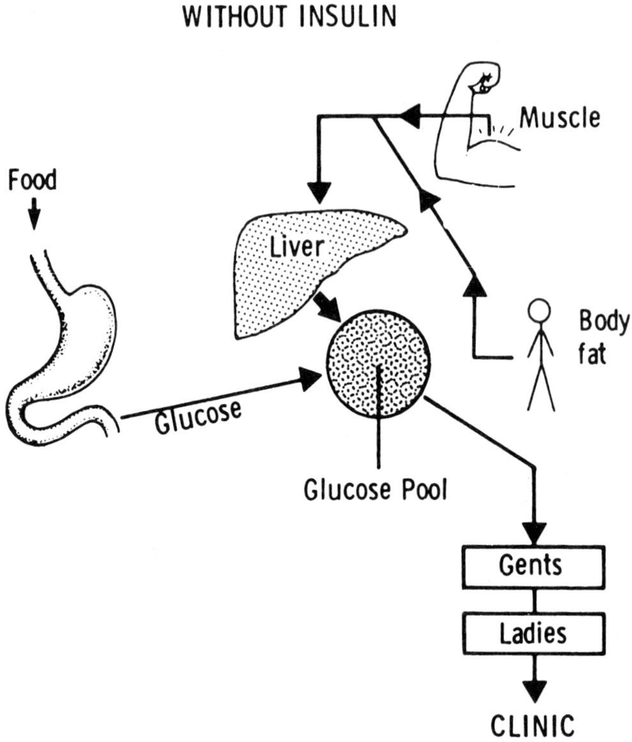

Fig. 1.4 Insulin deficiency. Without insulin, glucose cannot be stored so the glucose pool expands. At the same time, fat and muscle are broken down and changed by the liver to glucose. Eventually the glucose pool overflows and leads to excessive urination. (Reproduced with permission of Churchill Livingstone.)

Table 1.1 Common symptoms of diabetes

- Thirst
- Polyuria
- Nocturia
- Urgency or incontinence
- Balanitis or pruritis vulvae
- Blurred or misty vision
- Weight loss
- Lethargy

sufficient insulin is produced. Under these circumstances carbohydrate from food cannot be used efficiently and accumulates in the blood as glucose; shortage of insulin also allows glycogen, fat and protein to be broken down to glucose. Thus a high blood glucose level (*hyperglycaemia*) can develop even if the person is not eating. This causes loss of appetite, apathy and weakness. Overspill into the urine draws water, sodium and potassium out causing urinary frequency and thirst. Glucose in the urine encourages yeasts to grow on the skin causing irritation of the penis or vulva. Glucose also accumulates in the lens of the eye and causes misting or blurring of vision (a temporary phenomenon, not to be confused with diabetic retinopathy, see page 115). Breakdown of muscle protein causes weakness and wasting and breakdown of fat causes weight loss. Finally, if insulin supply fails altogether, the patient becomes ketotic with typical symptoms of shortness of breath, nausea and vomiting.

The symptoms experienced by an individual patient depend upon his age, how quickly diabetes has developed, how high the blood glucose is and whether he becomes ketoacidotic. Thirst and polyuria are almost invariable although, if diabetes develops slowly, the patient may be unaware of them; he may regard it as quite normal to have to drink pints of water through the day and get up three times at night to urinate!

CAUSES AND TYPES OF DIABETES

These are shown in Table 1.2.

Secondary diabetes

Just as Von Mering and Minkowski made dogs diabetic by pancreatectomy, destruction of the whole pancreas is one cause of diabetes in man. There is such a large reserve of insulin-producing cells that over 90% have to be destroyed before diabetes develops. Acute or chronic pancreatitis and carcinoma are the commonest diseases that physically destroy the pancreas. Secondary diabetes can also be caused by drugs that reduce insulin secretion from the β-cells. Diazoxide, sometimes used to control severe hypertension, is the most potent of these, but more commonly used diuretics and antihypertensives such as bendrofluazide and propranolol can also cause diabetes. Their effects are largely reversible so that blood

Table 1.2 Causes and types of diabetes

Idiopathic diabetes
Insulin-dependent (juvenile-onset or type 1)
Non-insulin-dependent (maturity-onset or type 2)
Gestational (see Chapter 5)
Secondary diabetes
Damage to or removal of the pancreas
pancreatitis
pancreatectomy
carcinoma of the pancreas
haemachromatosis
Drugs which reduce insulin secretion
thiazide diuretics
diazoxide
beta-blockers
Hormones which oppose the action of insulin
steroid therapy
acromegaly
Cushing's syndrome

glucose levels usually improve when they are stopped. *Haemachromatosis* is an uncommon cause of diabetes; sometimes called 'bronze diabetes' (after the characteristic discoloration of the skin), it is due to excessive absorption of iron from the gut and deposition in the pancreas (as well as other hormone-producing glands, the heart and liver). Haemachromatosis rarely affects women.

Another cause of diabetes is overactivity of other endocrine glands. Growth hormone-secreting tumours of the pituitary cause acromegaly and, since growth hormone opposes the action of insulin, about 20% of acromegalics have diabetes. Similarly Cushing's syndrome (overproduction of cortisol due to a pituitary or adrenal tumour) is commonly complicated by diabetes because cortisol too is an insulin antagonist. Cushing's syndrome is relatively rare, but steroid treatment is common and one of the commonest causes of secondary diabetes.

Secondary diabetes has been discussed before idiopathic diabetes, not because it is more common (in fact it is *less* common) but because reversible factors have to be sought in every new case. In the vast majority, none can be found and the diagnosis is one of the two types of 'idiopathic' diabetes.

Table 1.3 Features of insulin-dependent diabetes mellitus (IDDM) and non-insulin-dependent diabetes mellitus (NIDDM)

	IDDM	*NIDDM*
Other names	Juvenile onset type 1	Maturity onset type 2
Age of onset	Usually less than 30	Usually over 40
Weight	Usually normal or underweight	Usually overweight
Prone to ketosis	Yes	No
Onset	Usually over weeks	Often over months or years

Insulin-dependent and non-insulin-dependent diabetes mellitus (IDDM and NIDDM)

Table 1.3 implies that there is a very clear distinction between what have traditionally been called 'juvenile-onset' and 'maturity-onset' diabetes. The cardinal difference is in the need for insulin. In practice, however, life is not as simple as this; there are occasional patients who develop diabetes in childhood and never need insulin, while others develop typical 'juvenile-onset diabetes' in their 80s! Today the terms 'insulin-dependent' and 'non-insulin-dependent' diabetes are generally accepted, more descriptive than 'type 1' and 'type 2', and preferable to 'juvenile-onset' and 'maturity-onset' because they make no assumptions about age. This chapter describes typical examples of these two ends of the spectrum, but the reader must appreciate that there are many patients who do not fit neatly into either category.

Insulin-dependent diabetes mellitus (*IDDM*)

This is an 'autoimmune' disease in which, like Addison's disease, pernicious anaemia and some types of thyroid disease, the body mistakenly targets its defence mechanism against its *own* cells; lymphocytes and/or antibodies destroy the β-cells but leave the rest of the pancreas intact. What triggers off this reaction is unknown but virus infections have long been regarded as a possible culprit. In rare cases, a virus infection may *directly* destroy the β-cells but this is the exception rather than the rule. Microscopic examination of the pancreas shows the insulin-producing cells literally engulfed by the killer lymphocytes.

Damage to the pancreas probably starts months or years earlier but causes no symptoms until, when over 90% of the β-cells have been destroyed, diabetes develops. The symptoms may develop extremely rapidly, particularly if a stress such as an infection increases the demand for insulin. Ketones in the blood and urine are the hallmark of insulin-dependent diabetes and indicate that insulin supply is severely compromised. Ketoacidosis (see page 64) is the most extreme manifestation of insulin-dependence. Before they develop diabetes, people with IDDM are no fatter or thinner than the general population. However, they often lose weight fairly rapidly and are therefore thin when the diagnosis is made.

Although insulin-dependent diabetes can present at any age, three-quarters of patients develop it before the age of 30, and over 90% of people who develop diabetes before the age of 30 are insulin-dependent. The peak incidence is in the mid-teens but it may be diagnosed as early as the first year of life.

Non-insulin-dependent diabetes (*NIDDM*)

Most people developing diabetes after age 40 can be treated with either tablets or a diet alone. The cause of NIDDM is even less well understood than IDDM but the β-cells seem to lose their ability to recognise a rise in blood glucose and respond to it by secreting insulin (a faulty thermostat). Strangely, they may be able to secrete insulin quite normally when stimulated in other ways. NIDDM is not an autoimmune disease and the pancreas looks relatively normal under the microscope. The primary difference from IDDM is that the pancreas still continues to produce some insulin, enough to prevent ketosis but not enough to prevent hyperglycaemia. Of patients with NIDDM 80% are overweight but 20% are normal weight or thin. Obesity causes diabetes by increasing the demand for insulin beyond the capacity of the pancreas to supply it.

The symptoms of non-insulin-dependent diabetes usually develop over weeks or months or there may be none at all; not uncommonly, glucose in the urine is a chance finding at a works medical or life insurance examination. About a half of newly diagnosed non-insulin-dependent diabetics are on treatment for hypertension; because they reduce insulin production, many commonly used antihypertensive drugs can precipitate diabetes in a person predisposed to it.

One situation which deserves special mention is gestational diabetes (see page 106). Like obesity, pregnancy increases the demand for insulin and may 'find out' the person who is likely to develop diabetes in later life. Although diabetes usually clears up when the baby is born, one in two gestational diabetics develop permanent, usually non-insulin-dependent, diabetes within 10 years.

The grey area between IDDM and NIDDM

Some clinics have the facility to measure islet-cell antibodies, a marker of autoimmune damage to the pancreas. A positive result strongly predicts insulin-dependence but, unfortunately, a negative result is unhelpful. In practice, the decision to use insulin is almost invariably made on clinical grounds. Ketonuria or ketoacidosis are the hard and fast signs of IDDM but there are other reasons why insulin may be given. It may be started unnecessarily. It may be used to control diabetic symptoms or high blood glucose levels which have persisted despite treatment with oral hypoglycaemics, often in people who are overweight and unwilling to diet but are not 'ketosis-prone'. Deciding whether or not someone is truly 'insulin-dependent' becomes important if there is a question of stopping insulin. The following features strongly suggest insulin-dependence:

- History of ketoacidosis or more than a trace of ketonuria at diagnosis.
- Onset of diabetes before the age of 30.
- Normal weight or underweight at the time insulin is started.
- Insulin started within a year of the diagnosis of diabetes, usually because of continued weight loss and tiredness.

Sometimes the only way to tell is by stopping insulin, monitoring the urine for ketones, measuring blood glucose and watching for symptoms of poor control. 'Once on insulin, always on insulin' is a popular misconception; while this is obviously true of those with insulin-dependent diabetes, some patients in the grey area can be given a trial of insulin to see if it benefits them which can safely be stopped if it does not.

HOW COMMON IS DIABETES?

Diabetes is one of the commonest chronic diseases. There are striking differences in its frequency between racial groups, the highest of all being in the Pacific island of Nauru where nearly one in two have NIDDM. Like some tribes of American Indians with a high frequency of diabetes (for example, the Pima), the Naurans have adopted a western diet and lazy lifestyle relatively recently and many are grossly overweight; in evolutionary terms, the pancreas has not kept pace with the increased demand for insulin which obesity imposes. In the United Kingdom, a recent survey in Southall (an area with a large immigrant population) found that NIDDM was over ten times commoner in Asians than Caucasians of the same age, whereas IDDM was scarcer. Classical IDDM is relatively uncommon in many African races and a form of diabetes unknown in more affluent countries (*tropical malnutrition type diabetes*) accounts for most diabetic patients in these countries. Because of such great geographical variation, it is impossible to generalise about the overall frequency of diabetes. However, surveys of whites in both the United Kingdom and United States have found that around 2% of the population have diabetes and about one in six of these have IDDM. In general, the older you are, the more likely you are to have diabetes, although you are relatively unlikely to develop IDDM after 60.

Is diabetes becoming more common?

It is often hard to tell whether diseases are really becoming more common or whether they are just being recognised and reported more frequently. However, there is good evidence that IDDM is on the increase. The same is true of NIDDM, partly because people are fatter than they were 40 years ago and partly because the elderly population (the age group in whom diabetes is most common) is expanding.

IS DIABETES INHERITED?

Unravelling the inheritance of diabetes was once described as 'the geneticist's nightmare'. Neither IDDM nor NIDDM are heritable in the same clearcut way as haemophilia, for example, but both have a tendency to run in families, NIDDM to a greater extent

Table 1.4 The risks of relatives of someone with NIDDM or IDDM developing the same type of diabetes

	NIDDM	*IDDM*
One parent diabetic	50%	2–6%
Both parents diabetic	80% or higher	Unknown
Brother or sister diabetic	50%	10%
Identical twin diabetic	100%	30–40%

These figures can only be regarded as approximations

than IDDM. This question is particularly important to the brothers, sisters or children of a diabetic patient, and their risks are summarised in Table 1.4. The identical twin of a diabetic has the highest chances of all, which illustrates that inheritance plays a part in the development of the disease, since the two individuals are genetically identical.

DIAGNOSING DIABETES

Whatever may be difficult or confusing about diabetes, making the diagnosis is not (Table 1.5). Typical symptoms usually lead to a urine test. Glycosuria suggests diabetes but is not in itself diagnostic because glucose can occasionally spill into the urine of non-diabetics at normal blood sugar levels (*low renal threshold*). But if the fasting blood glucose level is above 7 mmol/l, the diagnosis is

Table 1.5 Diagnostic criteria for diabetes

	**Venous whole blood glucose concentration (mmol/l)*		
	Normal	*Impaired glucose tolerance*	*Diabetes mellitus*
Fasting	<6	<7	≥7
2 h after glucose	<7	7–10	≥10

* Slightly different criteria apply if capillary blood or plasma rather than whole blood glucose concentration is measured.

More commonly, a random blood glucose is measured; ve 10 mmol/l on two or more occasions are required to diabetes. If there is still doubt, a glucose tolerance test done. This involves measuring the blood glucose first on an empty stomach and then 2 h after drinking 75 g of glucose (taken as a solution such as Lucozade). The same criteria apply to the 2 h value as to the random blood glucose. A fasting value less than 7 mmol/l with a 2 h value between 7 and 10 mmol/l is described as *impaired glucose tolerance*, carrying a 50% risk of overt diabetes in later life. A 2 h value below 7 mmol/l is normal.

PRINCIPLES OF TREATMENT

Confronted with a newly diagnosed diabetic, the first step is to apply the principles discussed above (see pages 11 and 13) and decide whether or not they are insulin-dependent. If they are, insulin treatment should be started without delay because ketoacidosis may be imminent.

Insulin-dependent diabetes

Why injections?

Insulin-dependent diabetic patients produce little or no insulin of their own so the aim is to take over the function of the pancreas. Insulin is broken down by the enzymes of the stomach so it has to be given by injection. It is absorbed at a reasonably steady rate from the fatty tissue below the skin (*subcutaneous tissue*) which has a good blood supply and is readily accessible to a short fine needle, so this is where it is injected. Injection sites are discussed more fully in Chapter 5.

Types of insulin

Insulin preparations differ in two main respects: their length of action (short, medium or long-acting), and species (beef, pork or human). Until recently, most insulin used in Britain and North America was extracted from beef pancreas. Three of the 32 amino groups which make up the insulin molecule differ between beef and human insulin so the body's defence mechanisms can recognise it as 'foreign' and partially 'neutralise' it with antibodies. Pork insulin, differing in only one amino acid group, is now widely used in preference because it is less foreign and raises less of an antibody reaction. Within the last 8 years, human insulin has become available. This is not, as many people mistakenly believe, isolated from human pancreas but is manufactured in one of two ways: either the one amino acid which makes pork insulin differ from human insulin is chemically replaced, or the insulin molecule is directly synthesised by a genetic engineering technique. There is likely to be a major, possibly complete, shift from pork to human insulin over the next 5 years.

The insulin first prepared by Banting and Best and used exclusively for the next decade was soluble insulin. Lasting only 6 h, it had to be injected several times a day, usually before each main meal. Eventually ways were found to bind the insulin in complexes and slow its absorption so that it could be injected less often. These medium and long-acting insulins can be divided into those which use zinc to delay their absorption (semilente, lente and ultralente) and those which use protamine (isophane insulin). Protamine is a protein derived from salmon sperm. One preparation which uses both (protamine zinc insulin or PZI) is the longest acting of all but is now rarely used.

Table 1.6 summarises the different types of insulin. In practice, the times of onset and durations of action of the various preparations can only be regarded as generalisations because they differ from one person to another and from one injection to the next. Human insulin is absorbed slightly quicker and lasts for a shorter time than pork; beef insulin tends to have the longest action. Table 1.6 also shows several 'premixed' insulins which contain both soluble *and* isophane insulin.

Devising the ideal insulin regimen

Insulin treatment is a compromise between what is acceptable to the patient and what comes closest to the pattern of insulin secretion in the non-diabetic. The pancreas monitors blood glucose and gives appropriate amounts of insulin minute by minute, day and night; the artificial pancreas, a bulky piece of equipment controlled by a computer, works in the same way and has direct access to the blood stream through an intravenous cannula. Unfortunately, this form of treatment is extremely costly and is only practical for someone who is bedbound in hospital. However, impractical

Table 1.6 Types of insulins

	Peak (h)	Length of action (h)	Generic name	Species	Trade name
Short-acting	1–2	6	Soluble	Human	Human Actrapid
					Human Velosulin
					Humulin-S
				Pork	Velosulin
				Beef	Quicksol
					Neusulin
					Hypurin soluble
			Semilente	Pork	Semitard
Medium-acting	4–8	12–24	Isophane	Human	Humulin I
					Human Insulatard
					Protaphane
				Pork	Insulatard
				Beef	Neuphane
					Monophane
			Lente	Human	Humulin Zn
					Human Monotard
				Beef	Tempulin
					Neulente
Long-acting	8–12	24	Ultralente	Human	Ultratard
Pre-mixed insulins (soluble and isophane)				Human	Humulin M1 and M2
					Actraphane
					Mixtard
				Pork	Mixtard
					Initard

though it may be, the artificial pancreas illustrates the sort of insulin profile which needs to be supplied by an insulin regimen.

Figure 1.5 shows that a background trickle of insulin is required throughout the 24 h period, even during sleep. Surges of insulin after each meal or snack keep blood glucose within normal limits. Figure 1.5 also shows the principle of five commonly used insulin regimens. Once-daily long-acting insulin acts throughout the 24 h but does not reproduce the peaks and troughs. A mixture of short-acting and medium-acting insulin injected twice a day is better but has the major disadvantage that the evening medium-acting insulin, with a peak at about 6 h and a duration of approximately 12 h, may provide too much insulin during the night and wear off by breakfast time, causing the blood sugar to dip too low during sleep; that can be remedied by ‘splitting’ the evening injection, giving the short-acting on its own before the evening meal and the

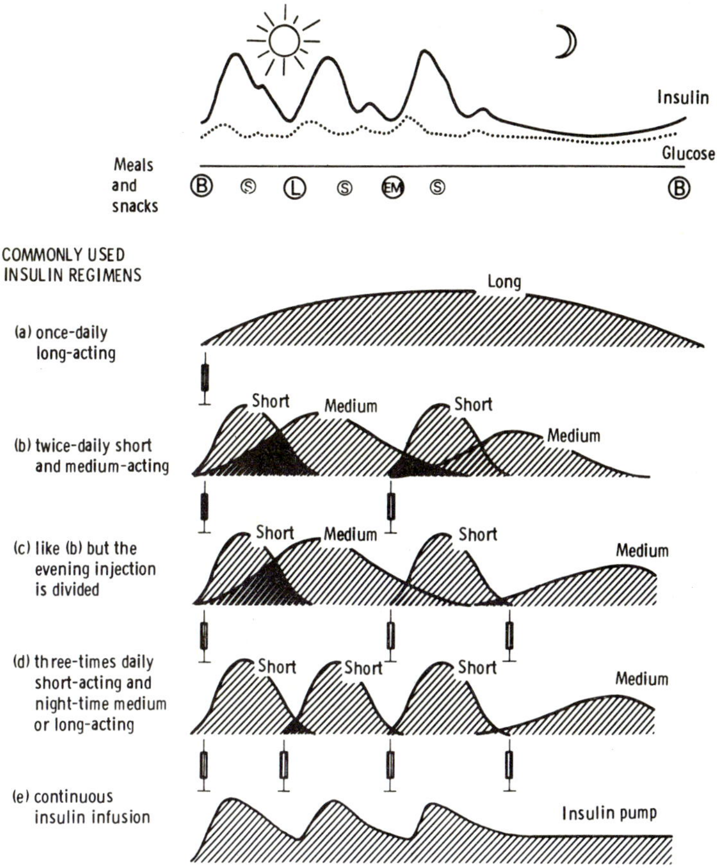

Fig. 1.5 The principle of five commonly used insulin regimens. Top panel: an artificial pancreas needs to produce a sharp surge of insulin after each meal and snack to maintain blood glucose within narrow limits; lower panels, five commonly used insulin regimens. (a) A single daily injection of long-acting insulin provides insulin throughout the 24 h but does not imitate the normal peaks and troughs. (b) Twice-daily short-acting and medium-acting insulin provides separate peaks of insulin action to cover the three main meals, and nighttime. (c) Similar to (b), but the evening medium-acting insulin is given immediately before bed—this more closely imitates overnight insulin supply in health. (d) Injections of short-acting insulin cover each of the three main meals; as in (c), an injection of medium-acting or long-acting insulin 'covers' nighttime. (e) Continuous insulin infusion from a portable pump. 'Pulses' of insulin are given before each main meal and a steady trickle continues through the night.

medium-acting last thing before bed. Even so, it is hard to regulate insulin supply during the daytime and meals and snacks may have to be 'eaten by the clock'. Injections of short-acting insulin before each meal provide greater flexibility with a dose of medium-acting or long-acting insulin to last through the night. Since each meal is matched to an insulin dose, this is particularly suitable for people whose mealtimes are very variable or who like to be able to alter the amount they eat at will.

Insulin infusion pumps, a new treatment, use short-acting insulin which is trickled through a plastic cannula or needle in the subcutaneous tissue, and extra doses are given at the press of a button before meals. Unfortunately, the pumps have to be worn on a belt or holster; most are larger than a pack of playing cards and may be a nuisance to carry around or uncomfortable to wear. Their other immediate disadvantage is that they cost upwards of £300. Other pros and cons are discussed on pages 131–5.

Diet and IDDM

Even the shortest-acting insulin lasts 6 h, whereas most carbohydrate is absorbed within 3 h so snacks between meals are usually needed to prevent blood glucose from dropping too low. In general, the more injections, the greater the flexibility in the timing and size of meals, but snacks may be needed even with a pump or four times/day insulin. Planning the diet for someone with IDDM is described in Chapter 5; the main principles are to:

- Adjust the calorie content to achieve and maintain ideal weight.
- Eat unrefined carbohydrate (starch or high fibre foods) rather than refined carbohydrate (sugar) to delay carbohydrate absorption.
- Keep the timing and amount of carbohydrate as constant as possible unless on a pump or 'multiple injection' regimen.
- Keep a balance between meals, insulin doses and exercise.

The balance between insulin, diet and exercise

Until now, no mention has been made of exercise, the third main factor that affects diabetic control (Fig. 1.6). Exercise can lower blood glucose both by 'burning it off' and also by increasing blood flow to the injection site and 'mobilising' insulin. Patients on insu-

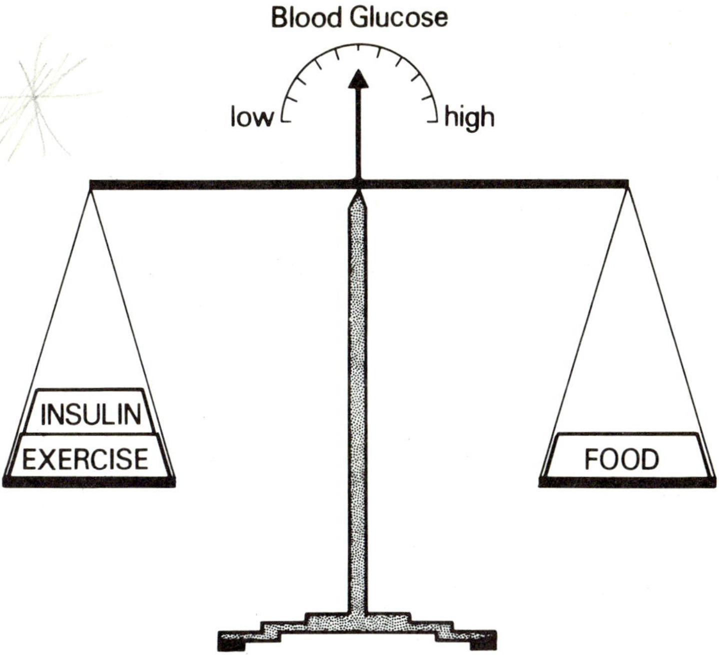

Fig. 1.6 Diabetic control is a balance between food (which raises blood sugar) and insulin and exercise (which lower it).

lin have to allow for this either by reducing their insulin dose or taking extra food before sports or other activities. In Chapter 4 this is discussed more fully, and examples are given of how it is done in practice. Whether during sports or everyday life, the balance between insulin, diet and activity has to be monitored; this is discussed below.

Hypoglycaemia

No insulin regimen is perfect, and blood glucose varies much more in people with insulin-dependent diabetes than in non-diabetics, sometimes completely unpredictably. Not surprisingly, blood glucose sometimes dips too low; this is called *hypoglycaemia*, and is defined as a blood glucose less than 2.5 mmol/l. It is discussed in Chapter 4.

Non-insulin-dependent diabetes (NIDDM)

Non-insulin-dependent differs from insulin-dependent diabetes in that the pancreas continues to produce some insulin, but not enough to control blood glucose, so the insulin must be made to go further. Most patients are overweight and, as a result, insulin-resistant so weight loss is the principal aim. Apart from being rich in calories, sugar causes a sharp increase in blood glucose which exhausts the flagging β-cells. Unrefined carbohydrate (preferably containing plenty of fibre) is more suitable whether the patient is thin or fat. Finally, if diet fails, tablets may be needed (see Case History 7.2, page 148).

Treatment

Oral hypoglycaemics fall into two classes, the sulphonylureas (such as tolbutamide, chlorpropamide, glibenclamide, gliclazide) and biguanides (metformin is the only one available in the United Kingdom). Both classes tend to reduce insulin resistance but sulphonylureas also boost insulin production. The major disadvantage of sulphonylureas is that they usually cause weight gain and can quickly undo all the good that has been done by months of conscientious dieting (page 148). They can also cause hypoglycaemia (see page 181). Metformin is less widely used than the sulphonylureas but has the great advantage that it favours weight loss rather than gain. It cannot cause hypoglycaemia and is the first-line drug for patients who remain obese and poorly controlled on diet alone, although side-effects sometimes limit its usefulness.

Insulin may be used to treat patients who are not insulin-dependent (as defined above) if their control is unsatisfactory on diet and/or tablets. The decision to treat with insulin in this situation is a matter of opinion and different doctors might choose to treat the same person with diet alone, with tablets or insulin. The proof of the pudding is not just the blood glucose levels and how the patient feels but, ultimately, which treatment is best at preventing complications. At present this is a matter for debate because no long-term research studies have provided definite answers.

MONITORING

As in any other disease, it is not good enough *just* to treat diabetes, there has to be some way of checking that the treatment is working. This is particularly important to people on insulin who need

Table 1.7 Methods of monitoring diabetes

- Symptoms of hyperglycaemia and hypoglycaemia
- Weight
- Urine glucose
- Blood glucose tests by doctor or nurse
- Home blood glucose monitoring (HBGM)
- Haemoglobin A_1 (HbA_1)

to adjust their insulin, diet and activity to keep themselves in balance throughout the day. The problem is that you can only *feel* changes in blood glucose when they are extreme and such feelings may be very unreliable. For example, people who are accustomed to running blood glucose levels five times as high as normal may feel terrible if their blood glucose is brought down to normal. If, as sometimes happens, they adjust their treatment to keep themselves feeling well, they will *always* have high blood sugar levels and will probably do themselves serious harm. Table 1.7 shows the ways of monitoring diabetic control. No single method is right for all patients and the choice will depend on the treatment objective in an individual case; there is no sense in frequently monitoring blood glucose or haemoglobin A_1 (see page 26) in an elderly person if the aim of treatment is simply to prevent diabetic symptoms and maintain body weight.

Weight

This index of diabetic control costs nothing to measure and is often forgotten but is an excellent indicator of well-being. Very poor diabetic control always causes weight loss; this may, for example, be an important clue that insulin is needed (see page 173). Similarly, 'overtreatment' with insulin (see page 98) or tablets (see Case History 7.2, page 148) usually causes weight gain.

Urine glucose

Urine testing is the time-honoured way of monitoring diabetes, and few patients escape without being taught how to do it, but how useful is it? The principle is straightforward: as blood glucose rises, a point is reached (*renal threshold*) when glucose spills over into the urine. With a further increase in blood glucose, the urine glucose concentration rises further still. This sounds simple enough, but it begs several questions. Is the renal threshold a fixed, unchanging level? Does the urine glucose concentration rise in parallel with blood glucose above the renal threshold? Does urine glucose accurately reflect blood glucose? The answer to each of these questions is 'No'. The renal threshold can vary from as low as 6 mmol/l in some, to as high as 15 mmol/l in the elderly, and urine glucose correlates poorly with blood glucose. Urine testing has other problems; whereas blood glucose changes from hour to hour during the day, the result of a urine test averages out all the glucose which has reached the bladder since it was last emptied. Worse still, because the renal threshold is often above 10 mmol/l, urine tests can give no information at all about blood glucose levels close to or within the normal range. This is a serious handicap when it comes to predicting or diagnosing hypoglycaemia; a urine test cannot be more negative than negative! Fig. 1.7 shows how poorly urine tests predict the blood glucose level at the same moment.

Much has been said about the shortcomings of urine testing but what are its strengths? Not everyone likes messing around with urine but, unlike blood, it is readily available. *Double voiding* (emptying the bladder twice in close succession so that the second sample contains fresh urine) makes the test more representative of the blood glucose concentration at the same moment. Urine testing comes into its own in older patients, particularly those not on insulin where the aim may be to relieve symptoms rather than to normalise blood glucose completely. Since many diabetic symptoms are caused by glucose spilling into the urine (see page 8), freedom from glycosuria may be an adequate indicator of successful treatment in older patients. Negative urine tests show that a symptom such as incontinence or urinary frequency is not due to poor diabetic control. Urine testing can also be used as a warning sign of diabetes going out of control; many older patients who have consistently negative urine tests can be told that strongly positive results, particularly if they appear during illness, should be reported immediately.

Blood glucose tests by doctor or nurse

A random blood glucose measurement in clinic or the general practitioner's surgery is another time-honoured index of diabetic control; like urine testing, it has shortcomings. It is quite possible to have a blood sugar of 16 mmol/l soon after breakfast and for it to be as low as 2 mmol/l before lunch. If the time relationship between the blood test and meals were standardised, the measure-

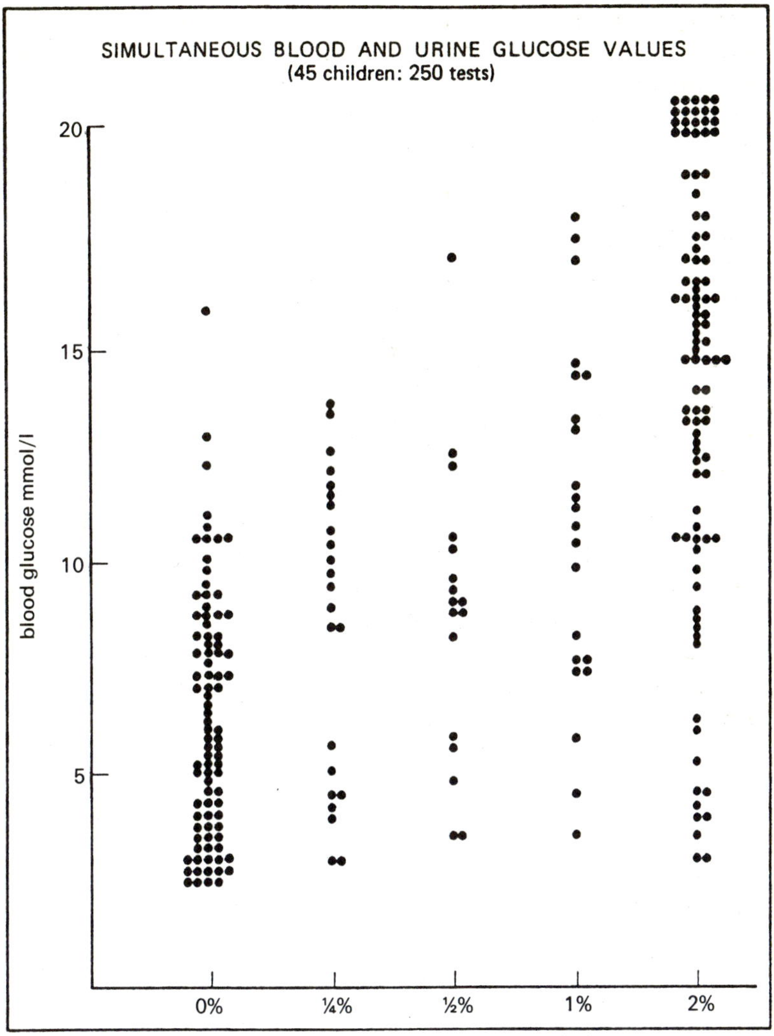

Fig. 1.7 This shows how poorly the urine and blood glucose concentrations correspond; someone who is verging on hypoglycaemia may have 2% glycosuria while others without glycosuria may be well over 10 mm l/l. Reprinted from Tattersall and Gale (1981), and reproduced with permission.

ment would be more valuable but this is rarely done. In insulin-treated patients it is risky to alter treatment on the basis of a single random blood glucose level because of its great variability. In NIDDM, the test can be made more informative by measuring the fasting blood glucose: this correlates well with blood glucose measurements at other times of the day and is the single cheapest and most informative test of control. Unfortunately, the same is not true in IDDM where fasting blood glucose varies unpredictably.

Home blood glucose monitoring (HBGM)

Home blood glucose monitoring has been one of the most useful innovations in diabetes care during the last ten years. At last patients can measure blood glucose directly rather than having to guess it from urine test results. The procedure is described in Appendix 5; in brief, a drop of capillary blood obtained by pricking a finger is placed on a reagent strip and left for 60 s. The strip is wiped with cottonwool and the result read 60 s later either by eye, comparing the strip with a colour chart, or with a battery-operated reflectance meter. For the squeamish, a springloaded finger-pricking device makes it easier to obtain the drop of blood; for the sanguine, a needle is all that is required. HBGM has many practical benefits; unlike urine tests, it can warn of imminent hypoglycaemia so blood glucose levels can safely be maintained close to or within the normal range when urine tests would be monotonously negative and completely uninformative. Also, unlike urine tests, the results do not lag behind changes in diabetic control so insulin doses and the size of meals can be calculated more accurately.

The main disadvantage is that a blood test strip costs three times as much as a urine test. But two tests can be had for the price of one by splitting the strip in two, and blood tests can give so much more useful information that the cost is generally justified. Whether the extra precision of a meter is worth while is largely a matter of personal preference. Strips read by eye are good enough for most situations although the extra accuracy may be needed in special situations like pregnancy. Visual readings make it easier for wishful thinking to affect the results, although it is not unknown for patients to deceive themselves and not write down their less flattering results even if they use a meter.

Haemoglobin A_1 (HbA_1) and fructosamine

Because blood glucose varies from hour to hour, the overall level of 'diabetic control' has always been difficult to measure. HBGM is one way of doing this, but not everyone is willing or able to do enough blood tests to give a full picture and those who do may 'improve' or even make up their results. What is needed is a test that accurately reflects average blood glucose levels over a period of weeks or months and is completely objective so that the clinic can have an independent index of diabetic control. Glucose very slowly sticks on to various proteins and the amount of glucose bound in this way depends on its average concentration in the blood. The most easily available protein is haemoglobin in the red blood cells and the amount of glucose bound to it can be measured. Haemoglobin A_1, the name given to this fraction of haemoglobin, averages blood glucose levels over a period of approximately 2 months. The concentration in non-diabetics is around 7% but most diabetics have considerably higher levels. Haemoglobin A_1 has now become the 'gold standard' for measuring diabetic control but one limitation must be appreciated: because it measures *average* blood sugar, a normal HbA_1 can be achieved either by consistently normal blood sugars or by swinging between high and low values. A 'good' HbA_1 may sometimes be a warning of recurrent hypoglycaemia.

Many hospital laboratories now measure fructosamine, the amount of glucose stuck onto plasma proteins rather than to haemoglobin. It is a cheaper test than HbA_1 but reflects blood glucose control over a shorter period (approximately 7–10 days).

THE IMPORTANCE OF SELF-REGULATION IN DIABETES

Diabetic patients are given a technically complex task and a responsibility for their own treatment which would daunt many professionals. Unfortunately, decisions have to be made when there is no doctor or nurse to hand and it is inevitable that patients and their families have to be in control. The task of the diabetes team is to give them the knowledge, self-confidence and support that they need to take on this responsibility but ultimately the patient has to be his own doctor.

FUTURE PERSPECTIVES

The aim of this book is to discuss the nitty gritty of diabetes care and theoretical information has been included at various points in the text to explain the practicalities. However, the last section of this chapter moves into the realm of theory and speculation, describing some of the areas in which future research may bring change.

Pancreas transplantation

Transplants are widely available for patients with kidney failure; in the best centres up to 90% 'take', and over half function for 5 years or more. Liver and heart transplants are often in the news, so why not transplantation of the pancreas? In fact, pancreas transplants *are* being done around the world including the United Kingdom but the success rate is still disappointing; even in the best hands, only one in three is working by the end of the first year. The pancreas produces not just insulin but potent digestive enzymes and 'drainage' of these enzymes has posed difficult technical problems. Solutions have been found but other problems remain: rejection of the graft may be difficult to detect and treat. If steroids are used, high doses are needed which may make the body more insulin-resistant and diabetes harder to control. Cyclosporin, a newer drug for rejection, is more effective and does not cause insulin resistance but the results are still disappointing. There is also a shortage of organs to transplant because, unlike kidneys, a donor has only one pancreas. Technical improvements and further advances in the treatment of rejection will probably improve results, but for the time being pancreas transplantation will usually be reserved for diabetic patients with renal failure who need kidney transplants and can receive a pancreatic graft at the same time.

A portable artificial pancreas

In this era of microprocessor technology, the hurdle of miniaturising a device which can take over the function of the pancreas does not sound insurmountable. Unfortunately, a glucose sensor which works reliably over long periods of time has not yet been developed and the implantable pancreas is far from becoming a reality.

Prevention of insulin-dependent diabetes

Prevention is better than a cure. With all the effort that has gone into investigating the causes of insulin-dependent diabetes, why is prevention not just around the corner? The most serious snag is that it is hard to predict who is likely to develop IDDM (Table 1.4

shows that the risks are not particularly high, even for first-degree relatives of someone with diabetes). If, for example, a vaccine were available, large numbers of people would have to be vaccinated to prevent disease in very few.

But what about treating the underlying cause rather than just putting the newly diagnosed diabetic onto insulin? By the time someone is found to have IDDM, damage to the pancreas is far advanced (at least 90% of the islets have been destroyed) and treatment at this stage is like shutting the stable door after the horse has bolted. In practice, researchers in Canada and France have been able to protect the few remaining islets for short periods of time with cyclosporin treatment. While patients continue to take this drug, they may be spared the need for insulin injections, but cyclosporin costs £1000 per year compared with £100 for insulin, has many side-effects and its long-term risks are unknown. It is feared that there may be an increased chance of cancer in later life, so its ill-effects may be worse than those of insulin.

Enough, then, of glimpsing into the future. For the present, diabetes is here to stay so the remainder of this book will look at the practical problems of people with diabetes and suggest some more mundane solutions.

Further reading

Bliss M. (1982) *The Discovery of Insulin*. Chicago: University of Chicago Press. The history of the discovery of insulin.

Bloom A., Ireland J. (1987) *A Colour Atlas of Diabetes*, 2nd edn. London: Wolfe Medical Publications. A colour atlas of diabetes and its complications.

Ireland J. T., Thompson W. S. T., Williamson J. (1980) *Diabetes Today. A Handbook for the Clinical Team*. London: HM & M. A practical guide to the medical management of diabetes.

Marble A., Krall L. P., Bradley R. F., Christlieb A. R., Soeldner J. S. (eds) (1985) *Joslin's Diabetes Mellitus*, 12th edn. Philadelphia: Lea and Febiger. A comprehensive reference textbook.

Tattersall R. B., Gale E. A. M. (1981) Patient self-monitoring of blood glucose and refinements of conventional insulin treatment. *American Journal of Medicine*; 70: 177–182. A practical guide to the medical management of diabetes.

Watkins P. J. (1983) *The ABC of Diabetes*. London: British Medical Journal Publications. A practical guide to the medical management of diabetes.

WHO (1985) *Diabetes Mellitus. World Health Organisation Technical Report Series, no 727*. Geneva: WHO. Diagnostic criteria and types of diabetes.

2/
The Diabetes Team

PROBLEMS IN THE CARE OF THE PERSON WITH DIABETES

Diabetes mellitus is unique among chronic diseases; it is common, the diagnosis is easy to make, treatment depends on a limited range of well-tried drugs, and yet it may demand more expertise of the people who suffer from it and the 'professionals' who look after them than almost any other chronic disease. Why is this? First, it runs a long course. Apart from gestational diabetes (see page 106), a person diagnosed diabetic will be diabetic for life—people who have been on insulin for 40 or 50 years are found in all diabetic clinics.

Second, the patient and his family play a more active part than in the management of most other diseases. This includes not only obvious matters like eating a suitable diet, monitoring diabetic control with blood or urine tests and adjusting insulin doses but also broader problems like choosing a suitable career, taking a responsible attitude towards driving and coping with diabetic complications. Diabetes makes it all the more important for people to choose a sensible lifestyle and avoid bad habits like smoking. The risk of hypoglycaemia (see page 77) makes the family's involvement especially important, because no matter how knowledgeable the patient, a hypoglycaemic attack can make him unable to help himself. Finally, in a far from ideal world, diabetics may themselves have to make sure that they receive regular medical and nursing care.

Not surprisingly, diabetes profoundly effects personal and family life. The person who develops it may feel that he is no longer 'a whole person'. His family may be angry because their life is disrupted and they have an unspoken fear of diabetic complications. These tensions are not confined to home. As with epilepsy, there is a stigma which makes people treat someone with diabetes 'differently', even if he is not on insulin. Employers may discrimi-

Table 2.1 What the person with diabetes needs from his carers

- Support and reassurance when diabetes is diagnosed and if problems crop up later on
- Education about diabetes and its management
- Effective treatment
- A way of monitoring the response to treatment
- Well-coordinated continuing care
- Prevention and treatment of complications

nate unfairly against people with diabetes and friends may stop inviting them out for meals. Such prejudice is all too often found among health care workers as well as the general public. For no good reason, dentists may be unwilling to treat a diabetic, and doctors and nurses may refuse to take responsibility for simple problems like immunisation. Worse still, the diabetic may get conflicting advice and not know whom to believe.

Against this background, the needs of the diabetic patient can be summarised as shown in Table 2.1. What do nurses have to offer and how do they fit into 'the diabetes team'?

THE TEAM

Figure 2.1 shows the range of people who may be involved.

Primary care

In Britain, symptoms usually take the patient first to a general practitioner who will sometimes diagnose and treat diabetes without seeking advice from hospital. The practice nurse, district nurse and health visitor may teach, provide support and look after complications like foot ulcers. Elderly people may be very dependent on the general practice team, particularly if they are blind or unable to draw up and inject insulin. The advice of a dietitian or chiropodist can sometimes be obtained without referring patients to a hospital clinic. Diabetic 'miniclinics' which provide treatment, education, dietary advice, and screening for complications are run in many practices and have the advantage over hospital clinics that they are closer to home, less daunting to the patient and often better run.

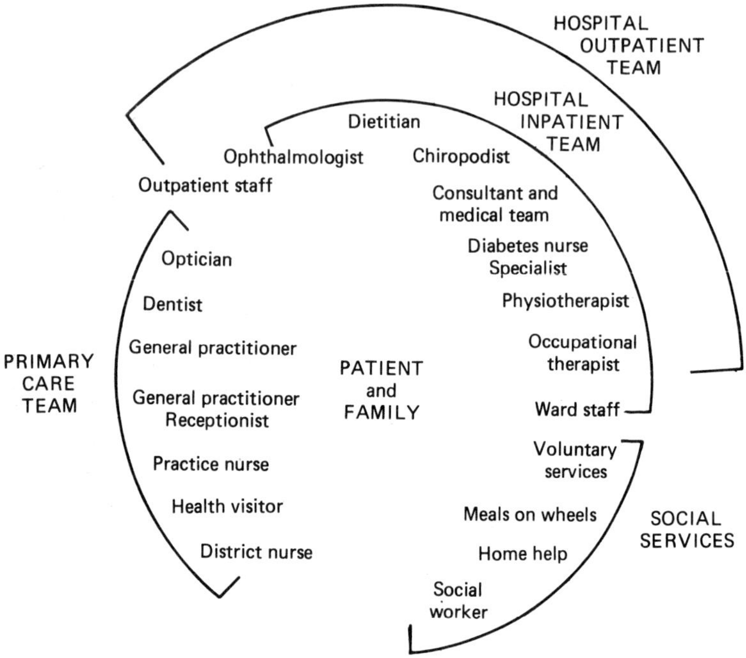

Fig. 2.1 The hospital and community workers that a diabetic patient may encounter.

The hospital team

Hospital referral is at the general practitioner's discretion; some refer all newly diagnosed diabetic patients, others only those on insulin or with complications needing specialised care. The referral may be to an ophthalmologist, a surgeon or a physician. Usually the consultant physician in the diabetic clinic is the first point of contact and he can refer on to other hospital departments if necessary. A dietitian and chiropodist attend most diabetic clinics, and other facilities such as physiotherapy, occupational therapy and social work can be called upon if necessary.

Admission to hospital for uncontrolled diabetes or complications may be arranged through the outpatient clinic or directly with the consultant or his junior staff. Many hospitals have one ward with a special interest in diabetes. The advantages of having a small group of nurses and doctors who are well practised at looking after ketoacidosis are obvious. As another example, the re-

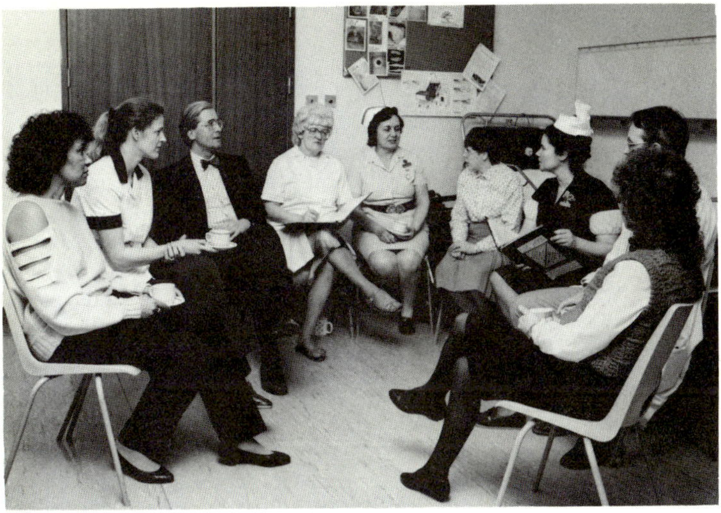

Fig. 2.2 A meeting of the diabetic team.

habilitation of amputees is best practised by nurses, doctors, physiotherapists, occupational therapists and social workers who are used to working together, interested and keen to get the best results.

Team meetings

For teams to work well, they need regular meetings to share ideas, discuss problems and maintain good communication. Figure 2.2 emphasises that these meetings should be multidisciplinary and relaxed, and that there should be no hierarchy because each member has equally important points to put forward. Having a good chairperson makes the meetings more productive. The members can take turns to do this to avoid domination by any one individual.

Overlapping roles and communication problems

At best, the 'extended team', illustrated in Fig. 2.1, can provide an excellent service but certain problems are common. Some members have no training in diabetes, communication may be poor and the roles of different members overlap, leaving the patient and his family confused in the middle (see Case History 2.1).

Case History 2.1

Mary is 35, has been on insulin for 20 years, and has had no advice about her diet since she was a teenager. She has an old diet sheet which restricts the amount of carbohydrate in her diet and forbids sugar. Her general practitioner arranges for her to see a community dietitian who allows her more carbohydrate but stresses that the timing and size of meals should be absolutely regular and that she must avoid sugar. The doctor also refers her to the hospital clinic where the diabetes nurse says that she can vary the amount and timing of her meals and eat sweet things provided she does frequent blood tests and adjusts her doses of insulin. Whom should she believe?

Doctors, nurses and dietitians may all give dietary advice and back it up with a diet sheet but there are different approaches and no single right answer. The mistake in Mary's case was that neither the dietitian nor the nurse realised that the other was advising her and neither gave an adequate explanation for the difference between their advice and her old diet sheet. This could have been avoided by better communication or by the general practitioner leaving her care entirely to the clinic.

THE PATIENT AND HIS FAMILY AS MEMBERS OF THE TEAM

Failure to recognise how much patients and their families know about diabetes is a common fault although their expertise is increasingly being recognised and exploited. Conflict may arise in hospital if the staff do not appreciate that treatment has to be tailored to the individual patient's needs and that he or she may have a better feel for it than they do (see Case History 2.2).

In this case, Jane knew best how to cope with her cold but, because she was 'only a patient', was not heeded. Even though she did not go into ketoacidosis and lose her baby, she lost all confidence in her doctors.

NURSES AS MEMBERS OF THE TEAM

A glance at Fig. 2.1 shows what opportunities there are for nurses to become involved in diabetes care at home, in the general practi-

> *Case History 2.2*
>
> Jane who has had insulin-dependent diabetes for 5 years and is 30 weeks pregnant is admitted to the antenatal ward for rest because of high blood pressure. While in hospital, she catches a cold. With her long experience, she anticipates that her diabetes will go out of control and knows that she needs to increase her insulin dose. The ward nurses cannot allow Jane to take extra insulin without a doctor's permission. The doctor on call is experienced in obstetrics but knows nothing about diabetes and insists on getting a physician's opinion the next day before altering her dose. Predictably, her diabetes goes haywire. Her anxiety about the effects of high blood sugar on her baby (see page 105) cancels out any possible benefits of bed rest.

tioner's surgery, in outpatient clinics or on the wards. Not only are nurses involved in every aspect of medical care but they are often better at getting on with worried people than other members of the team. Even the kindest doctor may be intimidating and slip into jargon which causes confusion and anxiety. A nurse sitting on the bed, chatting in the waiting room or calling at home may gain more insight into someone's problems after 15 minutes than a doctor achieves in 5 years of formal consultations. Apart from providing support and reassurance, nurses can play a unique role in coordinating the services provided by other members of the team (see Case Histories 2.3 and 2.4).

SPECIAL SKILLS OF THE DIABETES NURSE

Diabetes care is an ideal opportunity for nurses to adopt an 'extended role', either by taking more interest in diabetes as they encounter it in their own branch of nursing or by training as

> *Case History 2.3*
>
> It was not until the district nurse pointed it out that any of the eight other people looking after 81-year-old Miss Hardy (see Case History 8.2, page 173) realised she was attending the chiropodist, the ophthalmic clinic and the diabetic clinic in the same hospital on different days of the same week.

> *Case History 2.4*
>
> Mr Price has spent 8 weeks in a surgical ward with a foot ulcer. There is such pressure for beds that he is discharged home before the ulcer has healed and instructed to rest. Since he is 75 and lives alone this is only possible with the help of the social worker, general practitioner, district nurse, home help and meals on wheels. If these arrangements break down, he will start walking on the ulcer, 8 weeks' work will be undone in a few days and he may lose his leg. The ward nurses can make the arrangements when he first goes home but cannot follow his progress thereafter. A diabetes liaison sister can coordinate his treatment both in hospital and at home and follow him through until the ulcer is healed.

specialist diabetes nurses. The rest of this chapter examines the special skills in more detail and discusses why they are necessary and how they can be acquired. They can be summarised as follows:

- Good understanding.
- Authority to take decisions.
- Time.
- The ability to visit patients at home or at work.
- Teaching skills.

Good understanding

Sound practical ability, being able to give reliable advice and having the knack of anticipating problems are essential ingredients of good diabetes care. These come from a combination of experience, common sense and good theoretical understanding. A nurse working on a medical ward is too busy to master all the fine details of insulin treatment. On the other hand, a diabetes nurse specialist can devote more time to the nuts and bolts of insulin treatment and become better at it than all but the most specialised doctor. Good basic knowledge is essential for effective teaching; most people can spot nurses and doctors who do not know what they are talking about and will have no confidence in their advice.

Authority to take decisions

'Accountability' is one of the thorniest problems of specialised nursing. By tradition, it is the doctor's job to adjust treatment despite the fact that a nurse who knows the patient and has a good understanding of diabetes may be much better at it. Fear of legal action and the conservative attitude of the nursing profession make many nurses cautious about taking decisions. In Jane's Case History (2.1), the nurse's instinct was to allow the patient to adjust her own insulin doses but she correctly passed responsibility to the doctor. In practice, nurses with little understanding or experience are rarely foolish enough to take responsibility for 'medical' decisions. On the other hand, doctors who work with specialist nurses usually encourage them to make such decisions (after discussion, if necessary) and may include authority to alter insulin doses in their job descriptions. Complex tasks like management of foot ulcers are often best done jointly between several members of the team. Doctors who ignore the advice of an experienced nurse usually do so at their patients' expense!

Time and mobility

Of all commodities, time is one of the most important but scarcest. Take this as an example:

> *Case History 2.5*
>
> Mr and Mrs Bell have three teenage children. Mr Bell developed insulin-dependent diabetes 3 months ago and seems to have taken it badly. The diabetes nurse calls in at home one evening when the family are just finishing their meal. The eldest son remarks that the worst thing about his dad's diabetes is that mum never makes fruit pies or cakes any more and, as she is a super cook, he really misses them. Talking things over, it is obvious that the children resent their father's diabetes but no-one has ever discussed it with them. The diabetes nurse takes this opportunity to explain to the whole family what a diabetic diet means and how Mrs Bell can incorporate puddings into the carbohydrate allocation. However, it is obvious that more needs to be done to help them adjust to Mr Bell's diabetes. She arranges another visit when they will all be at home and gives them her telephone number so that they can contact her if fresh problems develop.

The nurse in this case has three important things to offer the Bells: she can visit them at home, take time to listen to their grumbles, and visit them again when they are all at home because her working hours are flexible. Making yourself available to diabetic patients and their families is a demanding but important part of the job. A nurse who gives her telephone number and offers advice and reassurance at the time when it is most needed gives a great sense of security to her patients.

Teaching skills

It has been repeatedly emphasised how much diabetes demands of the patient and his family. They have to learn new skills and be motivated enough to keep up their interests not just for the first 3 months but for the next 40 years. Each chapter of this book will emphasise the role of the nurse as a teacher. However, the ability to teach cannot be taken for granted and general training does not equip nurses with teaching skills. The diabetes educator has to learn how to fix realistic goals, bring home important messages by repeating them over and over again until they are fully understood and test performance and knowledge. The skill to teach effectively may come with experience but can be greatly enhanced by training.

The full-time diabetes nurse specialist

Whether in outpatients, on the wards or as a district nurse, 'non-specialists' are limited by all the other demands on their time. It should now be clear why there is a need for full-time diabetes nurse specialists who are not confined to a rigid schedule and can use their time flexibly and imaginatively as therapists, co-ordinators, confidants and teachers. Responsibility does not end

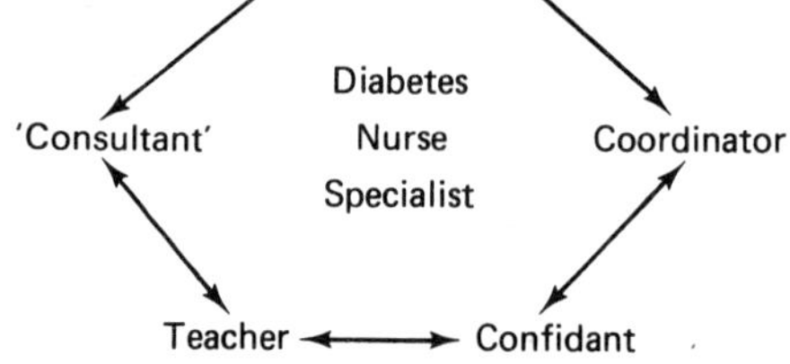

Fig. 2.3 The roles of the diabetes nurse specialist.

with the patient and his family. Specialist nurses can act as 'consultants' to other nurses, set up study days for hospital and community nurses and involve themselves in the training of student nurses, community nurses and health visitors. Figure 2.3 emphasises these roles.

COURSES AND TRAINING IN DIABETES NURSING

Both as an initial training and also to keep up to date with a fast-moving field, a number of training courses are provided for nurses.

English National Board (ENB) courses

These are run at various centres throughout the country. The formats of the courses vary and syllabuses are available from each training centre. Each school of nursing has a tutor responsible for ENB courses. Further details should be obtained from them or from the ENB National Office at Victory House, 170 Tottenham Court Road, London W1P 0HA (01-388-3131).

Diabetes Education Study Group courses

This group organises frequent multidisciplinary meetings. Further details can be obtained from: Dr John Day, Consultant Physician, The Ipswich Hospital, Heath Road Wing, Ipswich IP4 5PD.

British Diabetic Association

Within the Association are three sections which arrange meetings and act as a source of information: *Education Section:* yearly spring meeting lasting 2 days for all interested health professionals; *Medical and Scientific Section:* twice-yearly 2-day meetings predominantly devoted to scientific and research aspects; *Professional Services Section:* yearly meetings and study days for all health professionals.

Further details may be obtained from: The British Diabetic Association, 10 Queen Anne Street, London W1M 0BD (01-313-2351). In addition, the London office has professional advisers who can give advice over a range of matters related to diabetes.

Health Authority study days

Information about locally organised meetings can be obtained from consultant physicians with a specific interest in diabetes or diabetes specialist nurses. Other postgraduate courses in diabetes nursing are advertised in nursing and diabetes journals, available in hospital libraries.

The Royal College of Nursing has a special interest group for diabetes nurses. Details can be obtained from: The Royal College of Nursing, 20 Cavendish Square, London W1M 0AB (01-409-3333). Nurses wishing a more detailed training in teaching may take a course preparing them for the Adult Education City and Guilds 730 teachers' certificate available at colleges of further education. This is not specifically aimed at diabetes education but provides a useful groundwork for someone who is likely to spend the rest of her career teaching.

Health care is best practised by people who are conscientious and enthusiastic but know their limitations and are willing to learn. With that proviso, there is no reason why all nurses from the most junior to the most experienced should not make an active contribution to diabetes care.

Further reading

Kinson J., Nattrass M. (1984) *Caring for the Diabetic Patient*. Edinburgh: Churchill Livingstone. A textbook of diabetes for nurses.

Practical Diabetes (Asgard Publishing Co.). A periodical devoted to practical aspects of diabetes care.

3/

Diabetes in childhood

INTRODUCTION

Diabetes in a child means insulin and a diabetic diet for life. It is hard for the very young to understand why they are different from their brothers and sisters and are deprived of what they most enjoy eating, so every meal and injection may be a battle. Apart from coping with practicalities, parents often feel angry or guilty; 'why our child?' or 'have I brought this on by giving her too many sweet things to eat?'. They may feel that their child is no longer perfect. Blindness and gangrene may loom large in their minds every time she sneaks into the kitchen for a biscuit. Sympathetic handling of these psychological aspects as well as more mundane things like injections is the keynote, and the diabetes team should do all they can to encourage an optimistic view of the future.

Many aspects of diabetes in childhood are the same as in adult life so you will find frequent references to other chapters. These are the problems covered here:

- *Mary develops diabetes at the age of 4 and has to start insulin. Should this be in hospital or at home and what need her parents be taught?*

- *Paul starts truanting soon after moving up to comprehensive school; is he rebelling against school, his parents or diabetes?*

- *Mandy is 23 but severely handicapped with the mental age of an 8 year old. Her parents are struggling to cope with insulin and she is incontinent. What can be done to help them?*)

NEW DIABETES IN A CHILD

> *Case History 3.1(a)*
>
> Mary Jenner is 4. Her father is a lorry driver, her mother works part-time as manageress of a launderette, and she has a brother of 8. Mary goes to nursery school 3 days a week while her mother is out at work. For the last 3 weeks she has not been her usual self. Instead of being a lively chatterbox, she has lost interest in her toys and wants to sleep all the time. No amount of fluid will quench her thirst and she has gone back to wetting the bed at night. Her general practitioner recognises the symptoms of diabetes and finds glucose in her urine. He sends her straight to the hospital where she is admitted to start insulin treatment.

Starting insulin treatment in a child: hospital or home?

This is controversial; if the child is very drowsy, vomiting or severely dehydrated there is no decision to make because inpatient treatment is essential (other indications for hospital admission are shown in Table 5.1). In Mary's case the decision is harder. One could argue that taking her away from home at such a difficult time adds unnecessarily to her distress. On the other hand, her parents' needs must also be considered. Admitting her gives them a few days' breathing space and the hospital staff can help them to face up to their new responsibility. Nowadays parents are encouraged to visit as much as they like, and can usually sleep in, so hospitalisation need not separate them from their child. It has two other benefits: it allows the staff to teach the parents at a leisurely pace and gives them plenty of opportunity to ask questions. The Jenners may also find it supportive to meet other diabetic children and their parents.

Insulin can, however, be started at home if the right resources are available. An enthusiastic and well-informed doctor, district nurse or diabetes nurse can do this provided they have enough time to teach the parents how to give insulin injections, visit them repeatedly and make themselves available day and night for advice.

Both approaches have their virtues but the decision will ultimately depend upon local practice.

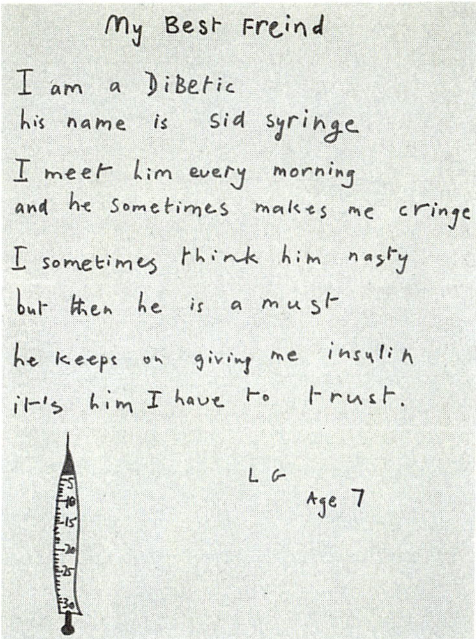

Fig. 3.1 Sid Syringe: a child's view of insulin injections.

Teaching the parents of a young diabetic child

Injections and insulin regimen

Technical details of drawing up and injecting insulin are covered in Chapter 5, pages 84–8 and Appendices 1 and 2. This discussion picks out important points for childhood diabetes. The first injection should be given as soon as possible so that the biggest hurdle is quickly overcome. One or other parent should be available to give each injection from the start. It is best for them not to draw up the insulin in front of Mary and to take turns giving the injections so that she will never blame just one of them for hurting her. Although parents know that it is for the child's well-being, they are very aware that they are inflicting pain with each injection. Unless they give themselves a dummy injection they will imagine it far more painful than it is. Injection time can be made less traumatic by devising games such as injecting teddy bears. In the last resort, parents may have to fall back on bribery by promising a treat.

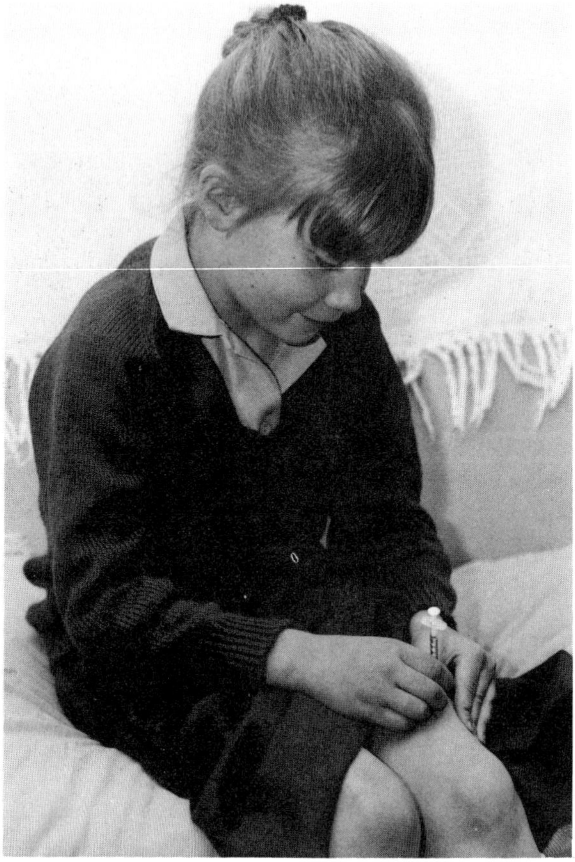

Fig. 3.2 Children may do their own injections as young as 5 or 6.

Whatever method is used, long confrontations should be avoided. Once it is clear that a child is going to refuse an injection, the parents should get on and do it. They should avoid giving all the injections at the same site or fatty lumps will form (*lipohypertrophy*, see page 89) which make insulin absorption unreliable. Children are wily so it is best not to let them find out that injections hurt less if they are always given in the same place—a habit which is hard to break later.

Different clinics favour different insulin regimens; some use once-daily long-acting insulin on the grounds that it is difficult to achieve good control in children with any regimen and you might

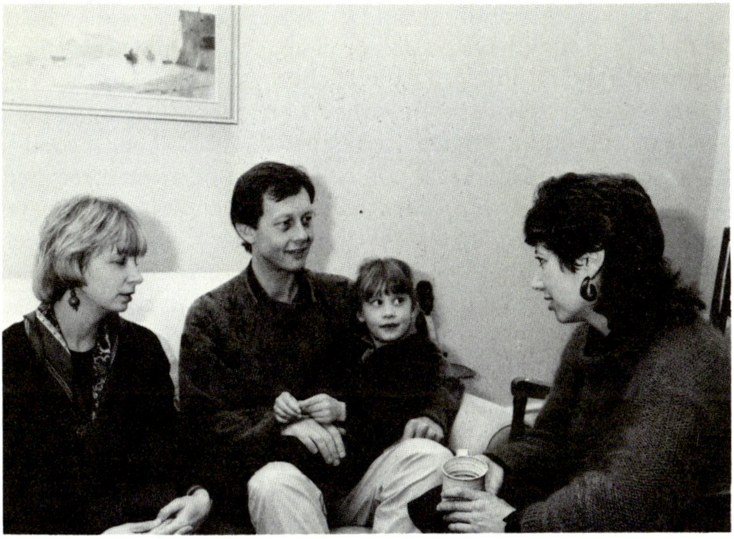

Fig. 3.3 A home visit by the diabetes nurse gives parents the opportunity to talk over the problems of their diabetic child.

as well minimise the number of injections. Others start with twice-daily medium-acting insulin; short-acting insulin can be added later but the parents have enough to learn at the start without the unnecessary complexity of mixing insulins.

Diet

Learning about the diet must wait until the parents are confident about giving the injections, perhaps the second or third day in hospital. Most clinics teach the *carbohydrate exchange system* to keep the amount and timing of carbohydrate as constant as possible (see page 93). Specimen plated meals, visual aids and a leaflet giving the 'values' of common foods help explain the system. A usual diet consists of three main meals with light snacks in between to prevent hypoglycaemia. The carbohydrate allowance may need to be increased when the child is more active at home and will certainly increase as she grows older.

Children's mealtimes can be a battle at the best of times and a great deal worse if they are not allowed the foods they would like. The diet of the diabetic child should be changed as little as possible and, ideally, all the family should eat the same. Unfortunately, the other children may have to accept changes which make them resent their diabetic sibling. Diabetic children soon learn that their parents worry if they do not eat their portions. This is the time to be patient and find an alternative rather than to argue. If food refusal is a regular problem, the injections can be given after meals and doses adjusted according to how much has been eaten. Restricting sweets is often the parents' biggest problem; special diabetic foods are unsatisfactory because they are expensive, and sorbitol, the sweetener used in most of them, can cause stomach cramps and diarrhoea. It is better to allow moderate amounts of normal sweets but count them as part of the carbohydrate allowance. As an example, at Easter it is better for Mary's parents to give her an Easter egg and let her have small pieces in place of desserts than to make her feel different from her brother or, worse still, to give neither of them an Easter egg and make them both resentful.

Monitoring

No two days are the same in a child's life; one day they may play indoors and watch television, the next they are sledging and snowballing. For Mary's parents the hardest task will be to balance her insulin doses and diet with these changes in activity. Some of the pros and cons of urine and blood testing have been discussed in Chapter 1 and practical details are given in Appendices 4 and 5. Many parents find that blood glucose monitoring gives them so much more useful information than urine testing that the extra discomfort is worthwhile. A finger-pricking device like the Autolet (one of several available) makes it easier to obtain a drop of blood. Different places should be used on different occasions and toes may be easier than fingers in struggling babies. At least one test each day, varying the time, and a 'profile' of two to four tests on 2 days a week is a suitable routine. The best times to test are before breakfast, before lunch, before tea and before bed. Extra tests can be done if the child seems unwell, has been unusually active or if her parents want to alter the size of a meal.

Hypoglycaemia

The thought of sudden unconsciousness is particularly frightening to parents. Many worry that their child will die during a hypoglycaemic coma (*hypo*), particularly if it happens during the night. They must be reassured that hypos *rarely have any lasting ill-effects*, but need to know how to recognise and prevent them (see Case History 4.4). Fretfulness, sleepiness or bad temper may be the only signs of daytime hypoglycaemia in a child of Mary's age; she may know that something is wrong without knowing if she is hypoglycaemic or hyperglycaemic. Nocturnal hypoglycaemia may cause restlessness or the child may wake screaming, as if she had had a nightmare. This can be very frightening to the parents.

The best way of treating a hypo is with a sugary drink (such as Lucozade), treacle or a proprietary glucose syrup which can be squirted onto the tongue or into the cheek (Hypostop), or a glucose tablet. Whatever difficulties there may be in recognising hypoglycaemia, both parents should carry glucose at all times because the ultimate way of deciding is to see what effect it has. However, they have to beware that their child is not claiming to be hypoglycaemic just to get glucose tablets or sweets. They should also both learn how to give a glucagon injection (Appendix 6) and always have it available at home.

Some hospitals deliberately induce a hypo to show the parents what they are like. This may allay their anxieties but can frighten the child. If it is done, the parents must be warned that hypos are not all the same and that the symptoms may be different next time.

The child's reaction to diabetes

A child of Mary's age will probably not be able to voice her feelings but a kind and sympathetic approach will help her. There is no reason to talk over her head or exclude her from discussions. It may be hard to explain the treatment but there are story books written specifically for diabetic children (see page 57). Her brother should be given a copy as well so that he does not feel left out.

Setting educational objectives

Before Mary is discharged, the diabetes team must be sure that they have taught her parents all the basics, the 'first aid learning objectives' summarised in Table 3.1.

Table 3.1 'First aid' learning objectives for the parents of a newly diagnosed insulin-dependent child discharged from hospital

	Parents should
Monitoring	be able to carry out blood or urine tests, record the results, know how to act upon them and how to test the urine for ketones during illness
Injections	be able to draw up and inject insulin, know the importance of varying injections sites and how to store and dispose of syringes and insulin bottles
Hypoglycaemia	know how to recognise the symptoms of both mild and severe hypoglycaemia and understand its causes, prevention and treatment. They and the child should carry glucose at all times and identification that she is diabetic (for example, SOS Talisman bracelet or necklace)
Diet	know why meals and snacks need to be punctual, why there is a need for carbohydrate exchanges and the quantity and type of carbohydrate in each meal and snack
Illness	know what to do in the event of childhood illness (such as measles) or vomiting
Nursery or school	have visited school and discussed diabetes with the teachers
Contact	know who to contact in times of crisis

Support after discharge

Case History 3.1(b)
Three days after admission, Mary is looking perky again and ready to go home. Her parents are given both the ward and the diabetes nurse's telephone numbers and urged to ring day or night if they need advice. Mrs Jenner's main concern is that Mary will refuse a snack at her nursery and go hypo.

Returning to nursery or school

Often the teachers are even more apprehensive than the parents. A visit by the diabetes nurse to explain the need for regular snacks and extra carbohydrate before exercise and to answer queries is time well spent. An information pack available from the British Diabetic Association provides useful information for schools. A lunchbox containing foods which the parents know the child likes is the best way of ensuring that she eats regularly. Parents should be encouraged not to keep her away from school because of diabetes or this may be the first step to problems with school attendance later.

Regular contact with the clinic nurse

A home visit within 2 days of discharge and frequent contact over the following weeks will boost the parents' confidence. A visit to the health centre allows the diabetes nurse to meet the general practitioner and health visitor, discuss Mary's progress and make sure that different people are not giving different advice.

Parents' support groups

One role of clinics is to introduce people like the Jenners to the parents of other diabetic children and many run parents' support groups. At best, these provide excellent practical advice and encouragement although experienced parents may intimidate those who are facing diabetes for the first time. Clinic nurses can introduce parents to one another although it is a matter of judgement whether this will be constructive and who would be suitable.

SCHOOL TRUANCY

Case History 3.2.(a)

Paul is a pleasant lad of 11 who has been diabetic since he was 6. Contact between him and the clinic has been limited to 4-monthly visits with his mother and father and occasional phone calls for advice. Last year, his mother was still giving his injections and taking all the responsibility for his diabetes so the clinic nurse suggested he should go to a British Diabetic Association summer camp. He learned about carbohydrate exchanges at the camp and started giving his own injections, to his mother's delight. Then 6 months ago he started at comprehensive school. At first he seemed to be enjoying himself, but his mother has just had a phone call to say that he has been truanting. Paul's parents are furious and there is a monumental family row after which Paul refuses to eat his tea and has a hypo. His mother rings the clinic to ask for an early appointment.

Truancy: naughtiness or a symptom of diabetes?

Truancy would not usually be regarded as a 'medical' problem, but it is a good example of how a chronic disease can affect the behaviour of a child and his family. It is not surprising that they should turn to the diabetes team for help. Here is how the team might respond.

Paul's mother probably expects the doctor or nurse to solve the problem by giving him a good telling off. This would only alienate Paul and give him a hostile doctor and nurse to contend with as well as angry parents, causing even more rebellion. Hearing why they have made an early appointment and knowing the family, these thoughts go through the nurse's mind: by truanting, he is consciously or unconsciously trying to make a point, presumably about a problem at home or school; of course, it may not be related to diabetes but there have been so many changes in Paul's life recently that she should at least explore how these have affected him.

Case History 3.2(b)

Paul and his mother are seen jointly by the doctor and nurse at the end of clinic to allow plenty of time. It is a stormy consultation, but these seem to be the problems: since going to camp and starting comprehensive school, Paul has begun to taste independence; however, he has found it difficult to adjust to school because diabetes has made him feel 'different'. His way out has been to truant. On the positive side, Paul is interested in learning more about diabetes. The doctor compliments Paul's parents on all they have done in the past and explains that they must now learn to take more of a back seat. Paul must certainly learn more about diabetes so that he can take responsibility for it; greater self-reliance will make him feel less of an outsider at school. The plan, then, is for the nurse to:

- Visit Paul's parents to counsel them further.
- See Paul on his own.
- Visit the school.
- Encourage him to talk to his friends about diabetes.

Counselling

PAUL'S PARENTS
The nurse visits his mother and father at home during school hours and talks over a cup of coffee about Paul's difficulties. Obviously he cannot take full responsibility for his diabetes immediately but his parents must start to let go of the strings. They must allow him to learn by his mistakes, without saying 'I told you so'. More independence at this stage will help him through adolescence.

SEEING PAUL ON HIS OWN
During weekly meetings, the nurse gets a better idea of what has happened. In his previous school, the teachers had a more relaxed approach to diabetes. Since leaving, he has found how little he really knows about it and cannot cope with the anxieties of his teachers and friends.

VISITING THE SCHOOL
The nurse sees the teachers and identifies a number of practical problems.

Problems at school related to diabetes

In general, there are six main areas of difficulty, listed in Table 3.2, and illustrated in Case History 3.2(c), with possible solutions.

To dismiss truancy or other behaviour problems at school as naughtiness will not solve the problem. Much more can be gained by scratching below the surface, teaching and supporting the child and his parents and doing some discreet work behind the scenes at school.

Case History 3.2(c)

TEACHERS
Because they know little about diabetes, the teachers repeatedly ask Paul if he is all right, drawing attention to him and making his classmates think he will collapse at any minute. The nurse explains that he gets good warning of hypos and is most unlikely to lose consciousness but may sometimes need a glucose tablet during lessons. She tells them what they should do if he has a severe hypo, and leaves them the British Diabetic Association Schools' Information Pack. She asks the teachers to play down his diabetes and gives them her telephone number for advice about specific problems such as school trips. The more he can be treated like his classmates the better.

SCHOOL MEALS

Paul has been taking sandwiches for lunch while his friends go to the canteen. This is because the sittings are staggered and his mother is afraid that he will go hypo if he is on the late sitting. To make him a special case and always include him in the early sitting is one solution but will inevitably draw attention to him. A larger mid-morning snack on days when he is on the late sitting will prevent hypoglycaemia and allow him to do just the same as his mates.

SNACKS

Until now, Paul has been eating his morning snack in class because school break is at 10.30 and his routine is to have a sandwich at 10 am. This is the sort of routine which parents are afraid to break but may be completely unnecessary. The nurse sets Paul the task of finding out if he really needs snacks by doing blood tests on days when he does and does not have them. He finds that he can safely leave out his mid-afternoon snack but his blood glucose is low before lunch if he leaves out his elevenses; however, he can safely wait until break time at 10.30.

SPORT

Paul knows that he should take extra carbohydrate before exercise but does not know how much. He has not been allowed to take part in vigorous sports such as swimming and cross-country running because the PE teacher is worried that something dreadful will happen. The nurse explains that many professional sportsmen have diabetes and tells Paul how he can use blood tests to judge how much extra carbohydrate he needs (see page 72).

DETENTION

Some of Paul's friends have been kept late or have had to miss their lunch breaks for misbehaving. Paul's mother lives in fear that he will have a hypo if this happens. She is advised to ask the teachers to give Paul advance warning of detentions so that he can take the appropriate action.

TELLING HIS FRIENDS ABOUT DIABETES

Until now, his friends have only heard about diabetes from the teachers and Paul has been too shy to discuss it. He is encouraged to get them interested by showing them how he measures his blood glucose and give an injection. *He* rather than the teachers should tell them about hypos and explain that they do not cause permanent harm. He invites some friends round for tea so they can see that his home life is no different from theirs.

Table 3.2 Problems for diabetic children at school

- The attitudes and knowledge of the teachers
- School meals
- Snacks
- Sport
- Detentions
- Relations with friends and classmates

MENTAL HANDICAP

Case History 3.3(a)

Mandy is mentally handicapped. Although now 23, she has a mental age of 8 and can do nothing for herself. Her mother put a lot of effort into getting her dry at night and finally succeeded by restricting drinks and toileting her last thing at night. After Easter she started to wet the bed again and the strain was beginning to tell on her mother so her doctor arranged a relief admission to the mental handicap hospital. A routine urine sample was loaded with glucose. Mandy's mother was told that she had diabetes, that this was why she was wetting the bed and that treatment should help restore continence. During the 2 months in hospital she was treated first with tablets and then, because her diabetes was still poorly controlled, with insulin but her bedwetting did not improve. Now she is back home and, after a few visits from the district nurse, her mother is having to give her insulin injection each morning. She feels ill-prepared for this new responsibility and is at her wits' end because the bedwetting is no better.

This case history has been included in a chapter on 'diabetes in childhood' because it is Mandy's *mental* rather than her physical age that affects her management. It illustrates many points that apply to children and she will be referred to as 'a child' despite her age. Many of the points also apply to the other dependent age group, the elderly. It is not a coincidence that Mandy is both diabetic and mentally retarded: Down's syndrome (mongolism) and some other causes of mental retardation are associated with diabetes so most clinics have several patients like her on their books.

Mental handicap and diabetes: the aims of treatment

The mentally handicapped are often children of elderly parents and totally dependent on them. Already they may dominate much of their parents' time at the expense of their brothers and sisters. Their parents may worry about who will look after them when they die. It is difficult to generalise but a realistic aim in most cases is to use as simple a regimen as possible to control diabetic symptoms with the minimum possibility of hypoglycaemia.

Practical problems

Insulin treatment

Although the hospital staff did their best to keep things simple by treating Mandy with one insulin injection a day, they were wrong to believe that this would save her mother trouble. The morning injection of long-acting insulin is not lasting for 24 h and the blood glucose is rising overnight. As a result of this glucose is spilling into the urine, increasing the urine volume (*osmotic diuresis*) and causing wet beds. Attempting to overcome this by increasing the dose of insulin may be ineffective and cause hypoglycaemia during the day. Had the staff checked her urine, they would have found that she had negative tests in the afternoon and evening and heavy glycosuria before breakfast. If more effort had been put into teaching Mandy's mother how to give the injection, rather than relying on a daily visit from the district nurse, they would have found that she could manage perfectly well, that Mandy did not mind injections and that twice-daily insulin fitted easily into the family's routine.

The decision whether to start once or twice-daily insulin in the mentally handicapped and the elderly is largely determined by how well they are supported. However, even if there are practical problems about the second injection, the inconvenience may be more than offset by the benefits of improved control (dry beds, in Mandy's case). The only way to find out is by trial and error.

Diet

Mentally handicapped children tend to be very overweight and fond of their food. They often eat for comfort and mealtimes may be the highlights of their day. Imposing restrictions like cutting out sweet things may just cause tantrums. The general principles (which are much the same as in elderly insulin-treated diabetics, discussed in Chapter 8) are summarised in Table 3.3.

Table 3.3 General principles of diet in mental handicap

- A formal carbohydrate exchange diet is not usually necessary
- The diet should fit into family, school or work routine so far as possible
- Sweet things should be taken in moderation but it is best to avoid making this a point of conflict
- If the child is obese, avoid fattening foods and keep portions moderate
- Light snacks are usually necessary between the three main meals to prevent hypoglycaemia

Monitoring

The virtues of blood over urine monitoring are repeatedly stressed in this book. Paradoxically, in someone like Mandy (where the aim is to prevent polyuria and incontinence) urine testing has some advantages in that these symptoms are caused by glucose spilling over into the urine. If the problem is bedwetting at night, heavy glycosuria in the morning is a clue that diabetes is responsible. The main disadvantage of urine testing for parents like Mandy's is that it cannot help to predict and prevent hypoglycaemia. Ultimately, the choice will be a practical one. If Mandy's mother can only get a urine sample by squeezing out the drawsheet, then blood tests will be more convenient. If, on the other hand, finger-pricking causes tantrums, urine tests are preferable. If both methods present difficulties, it may be quite adequate to monitor control by occasional measurements of blood glucose or HbA_1. Finally, since the aim is to avoid both hyperglycaemic symptoms and hypoglycaemia, these alone can be used as the endpoints of treatment.

Hypoglycaemia

Hypoglycaemia adds an extra burden to the family caring for a handicapped child; however, variable activity and a less than rigid diet may make it hard to steer a middle course between hyperglycaemia and hypoglycaemia. Hypos may be hard to recognise; temper tantrums, sleepiness or fits are sometimes the only evidence. Regular meals and snacks and a suitable insulin regimen are the best ways of preventing hypos. Having a glucagon kit (see Appendix 6) for bad hypos which cannot be controlled with oral glucose will give the parents something to fall back on.

Psychological aspects

Parents of mentally handicapped children need a lot of support at the best of times. A physical illness like diabetes may intensify their guilt and insecurity. They are bound to worry about who will look after a totally dependent child after their death. They may be angry at having to cope with another problem in addition to mental handicap. The demands of their handicapped child may make them feel that they are neglecting their other children and they may find it hard to meet other parents in the same situation. The British Diabetic Association Welfare Department could help with the last of these problems by putting them in touch with someone in another part of the country whom they can telephone or correspond with.

Case History 3.3(b)

Regular visits from the district nurse give Mandy's mother more confidence in giving her injections and planning her diet. However, now that she is on insulin they have qualms about leaving her. They always used to take her younger sister to the social club for a game of bingo on a Saturday night, leaving Mandy in the care of a neighbour but they are not sure that they should still do this.

Babysitting and the child with diabetes

It is especially important for parents like Mandy's to go out for the evening with an easy conscience every now and then or they will resent their responsibilities even more. A sensible neighbour, relative or friend can quickly learn enough about diabetes to fill the

Table 3.4 Babysitting advice for the parents of a diabetic child

- Make sure that the babysitter knows how to recognise hypoglycaemia and what to do about it
- If hypos are frequent and unavoidable, teach the babysitter how to use a glucagon kit
- Try not to let the child sense your anxiety
- Check her blood glucose before going out so that you do not spend the evening fretting about hypos
- Leave a telephone number in case of problems

breach. It is ideal to have just one or a limited number of baby-sitters. Some other tips are given in Table 3.4.

Benefits and assistance for the mentally handicapped

Caring for someone like Mandy is not just tying but expensive. Some areas have specialist health visitors with responsibility for the mentally handicapped who can advise about financial benefits and local facilities for the handicapped and arrange holiday placements to give the parents a break. The diabetic clinic can help parents like Mandy's by contacting the health visitor and making sure that Mandy is receiving all the services and benefits available to her.

Further reading

Althea (1983) *I Have Diabetes*. Cambridge: Dinosaur Publications.
Rupert and his Friends. Ames Laboratories.
Educational material for young children.

Baum J. D., Kinmonth, A. L. (1985) *Care of the Child with Diabetes*. Edinburgh: Churchill Livingstone.
Farquhar J. W. (1981) *The Diabetic Child. Patient Handbook Series*. Edinburgh: Churchill Livingstone.
Textbooks of paediatric diabetes care.

4/

Diabetes in adolescence

UPHEAVAL AND REBELLION

This can be one of the hardest times of diabetic life, not only for the adolescent him(her)self but for his parents, nurses and doctors. Teenagers who become diabetic during childhood have their first real taste of independence in adolescence and may reject routine and discipline along with everything else which represents authority. Worse still, they may use diabetes as a weapon to manipulate their family or friends. A third to a half of all insulin-dependent diabetics are diagnosed between the ages of 10 and 20. A teenager suddenly confronted with insulin treatment for the rest of his life may angrily reject diabetes. This is not to say that *all* adolescents are difficult or poorly adjusted. Some adjust very well, but this is the time of life when it is hardest to come to terms with being 'different' and this must always be remembered when looking after adolescent diabetics. They demand patience, understanding and realistic goals. Four case histories will be discussed:

- *Susan is 14 and has been diabetic since childhood. She is repeatedly admitted to hospital in ketoacidosis. Why has a child with stable diabetes become a 'brittle' adolescent and what can be done to help her?*
- *Darren is an athletic 16-year-old who takes a pride in keeping himself well controlled. Can he run in the local marathon and how should he control his diabetes?*
- *Karen has just started as a student nurse and has always depended on her mother to make the decisions about her diabetes. How should she cope with shift work?*
- *Steven has a hypo in the pub and ends up in casualty. What is hypoglycaemia, what causes it and how can it be prevented?*

BRITTLE DIABETES

Case History 4.1(a)

Susan is 14 and has had diabetes since she was 8; she is an only child who lives with her parents. At first she had no major problems but over the last 2 years has had more than 20 admissions with ketoacidosis, so that a side ward is almost permanently reserved for her. She is away from school more often than she is there and her parents are distraught. Her insulin regimen has been changed repeatedly to no avail. Despite all Susan's admissions to hospital and visits to clinic, the problem is not improving. Her parents ask in desperation for a second opinion hoping that new people and a fresh approach may provide a solution.

What is 'brittle diabetes'?

This term is used to describe a person with insulin-dependent diabetes whose unpredictable swings between hypoglycaemia and hyperglycaemia prevent them from leading a normal life and/or result in repeated hospital admissions with hypoglycaemia, ketoacidosis or both. More often than not, brittle diabetics are teenage girls.

For Susan, it was ketoacidosis which brought her into hospital each time. Of course, ketoacidosis is not just a problem of brittle diabetes and can affect people of all ages, but it is highlighted particularly in Case History 4.1.

Causes of brittle diabetes

Table 4.1 lists the main factors which can cause such unstable diabetic control. 'Overtreatment' (see Case History 5.2, page 98), irregular patterns of diet, exercise and insulin, and other underlying disease should all be considered; there are also rare patients who do not absorb subcutaneous insulin and respond to it normally. However, it is striking how girls may go through a period of brittleness during adolescence and be quite stable in later years; such periods often coincide with stress or difficulty in their private

Table 4.1 Causes of brittle diabetes

• Inappropriately high insulin doses ('overtreatment')
• An irregular pattern of diet, exercise and insulin
• Underlying diseases
Infections
Cushing's syndrome
• Breakdown of insulin at the injection site
• Psychological factors
Carelessness
Deliberate omission or overdosage with insulin
Effects of physical or emotional stress on diabetic control

or family lives, underlining the psychosomatic origin in at least a proportion of cases.

Psychological aspects of brittle diabetes

Adolescence can involve stress and conflict at home, school and work. Diabetes gives the person who suffers from it a powerful weapon to get out of confrontations; taking extra insulin, missing a meal or omitting an injection can produce rapid and dramatic results which focus attention on the diabetic patient and attract sympathy. This manipulation is not necessarily deliberate, and may be a response to difficult situations over which the brittle diabetic otherwise has no control such as tension between her parents. Even in those who do not manipulate their treatment, stress can affect diabetic control by upsetting routine and increasing blood levels of the 'stress hormones' that oppose the effects of insulin (see page 64).

Effects of labelling someone 'a brittle diabetic'

When describing someone as 'brittle', it is important to remember the consequences this may have for them:

- They may feel that they are physiologically 'different' and stop trying to control their diabetes.
- Once labelled, doctors and nurses mistrust them and develop a sense of hopelessness, particularly if the case notes are more than 5 cm thick!
- Because they are regarded as 'lost causes', medical and nursing

staff may just deal with each new crisis as it arises rather than try to get to the root of the problem.

How to tackle the problem

For the clinic to which she is now referred, the options are to:

- Continue to deal with the crises of ketoacidosis and hope that all will settle down as she gets older.
- Concentrate on intensifying her insulin therapy, diet and monitoring.
- Search for organic causes of brittle diabetes.
- Seek evidence of manipulation.
- Build up a relationship with Susan and her family to find out how they interact and where the problems may lie.

The first option has already been tried and failed. Susan will continue to fall behind at school and forfeit her chances of a job later on so long as the problem continues, and one of her episodes of ketoacidosis might even be fatal. Her parents will become yet more anxious, they will be afraid to leave Susan alone and their own relationship will suffer. These family tensions can then perpetuate a vicious circle leading to further episodes of ketoacidosis. Somehow the cycle has to be broken. The second option is to admit her to hospital, measure numerous blood glucose profiles and try yet more types and doses of insulin. A pen injector or insulin infusion pump might be tried (see page 132). However, the many previous changes in insulin regimen have done no good, so unless the problem is gross overtreatment (in which case reducing the dose of insulin may solve the problem) why should this be any more successful?

Of course organic causes must be excluded; the diabetic should be examined by a competent physician, blood tests and a chest X-ray should be arranged and her temperature monitored if there is any suggestion of a febrile illness. The rare problem of insulin breakdown at the injection site can be excluded by comparing her response to subcutaneous and intravenous insulin. Unfortunately, these tests rarely provide an answer.

Brittle diabetes is all too often caused by deliberate manipulation which may be remarkably hard to prove, even in hospital. No method of insulin administration will foil the determined manipulator. Nurses should be aware of the possibility and keep their eyes open for such things as:

- Secret supplies of insulin, smuggled into hospital and hidden in a bedside locker, toilet cistern etc.
- Filling insulin bottles with water.
- Stealing extra insulin from ward stocks.
- Injecting insulin into the mattress rather than the thigh.

Some patients are never found out and only admit their misdeameanours in later years. Whether or not this is suspected or proven, what is even more important than spotting manipulation is to consider its cause. The fifth option, to build up a relationship with Susan and her parents and try to identify underlying problems, is the best bet in the long run. No two brittle diabetics are the same but, as an example, here is how Susan's case is tackled.

Case History 4.1(b)

First impressions suggest that there are serious problems within the family which may take some time to unravel. The immediate plan is to break the pattern of repeated admissions and time lost from school; getting to grips with what lies below the surface will probably take longer.

Immediate care

KEEP HER OUT OF HOSPITAL

The doctor and diabetes nurse visit Susan at home on a number of occasions to teach her parents how to recognise the early symptoms of ketoacidosis and abort the episodes. Vomiting is an early symptom which seems in her case to precede ketosis rather than be an effect of it. Her parents are taught how to control the vomiting with intramuscular metaclopramide and use blood tests and extra insulin doses to prevent ketosis. With plenty of home visits and a telephone number to ring for advice, they manage to abort some, but not all, episodes.

KEEP HER AT SCHOOL

She is losing time from school because she is sent home whenever she feels unwell. With the cooperation of the school nurse and teachers, support from the diabetes nurse and ready access to advice from the hospital by telephone, her vomiting and ketosis could be controlled at school as at home. After some initial resistance, Susan's parents are persuaded to trust the school nurse and let her go to school even when she feels unwell and does not want to go.

PROVIDE CONTINUING SUPPORT

Regular meetings between Susan's parents and the doctor, diabetes nurse, and school nurse stop them from losing heart even when the going is tough.

Having worked out a way to prevent ketoacidosis, the diabetes team have won the confidence of Susan's parents and bought time to get to the root of the problems and put some structure back into their lives.

Medium-term care

The doctor and diabetes nurse are experienced in family therapy; they arrange to meet Susan and her parents for an hour on a number of occasions to talk about their home situation rather than diabetes. From these sessions, this is the picture that emerges:

Susan's grandmother died of a chest complaint in their house 2 years ago. Susan is terrified that her mother, who has chronic bronchitis, will die as well and worries about who would then look after her diabetes. Understandably, she wants to stay at home to look after her mother. Although she has often cried about this in bed at night, she has never been able to tell anyone. This is made especially difficult because her father is the sort of person who tries to cheer people up rather than allow them to express their feelings. He demonstrates this during one of the family therapy sessions when Susan bursts into tears; this is an opportunity to point out that he should wait and find out why she is so sad. Susan's mother also has fears which she has not been able to express before.

The strength of this approach is that, once a family have aired their unspoken anxieties and can face up to them, there is no need to use diabetes to express them.

Long-term care

Susan's family are advised to set aside an hour at the same time each week specifically to talk to each other. At this stage the doctor and diabetes nurse have to keep in touch with the family but step into the background and wait to see how things turn out.

Whatever the outcome, the aim must be not to let Susan or her parents lose faith in the clinic. Unfortunately, this is not always how it works out. Some adolescents rebel and only return when they have begun to develop complications. More often than not, this is because the diabetes team never got to grips with their real problems and blamed rebellion on being a teenager rather than on their own lack of understanding.

KETOACIDOSIS AND NON-KETOTIC HYPER-OSMOLAR COMA

These terms describe hyperglycaemic emergencies in diabetic patients; page 170 discusses how to distinguish them from hypoglycaemia. Ketoacidosis can affect insulin-dependent diabetic patients of all ages, whereas hyperosmolar non-ketotic coma affects older patients, often with non-insulin-dependent diabetes. As the names indicate, the difference lies in whether or not ketones accumulate and the blood becomes acid (page 7). In practice, this does not make a great difference to treatment and the term 'hyperglycaemic coma' will be used here to describe both.

How does hyperglycaemic coma develop?

Maintenance of a normal blood glucose depends on the correct balance between insulin (which lowers it) and the 'stress hormones' (adrenaline, noradrenaline, glucagon, cortisol and growth hormone) which raise it. The balance is upset if there is insufficient insulin or increased stress hormones. A severe infection, for example, causes such an increase in stress hormone levels that hyperglycaemic coma can develop despite taking insulin doses which are usually adequate. In practice, hyperglycaemic coma is usually caused by a combination of events. For example, an attack of gastroenteritis puts a patient off his food. He is afraid of going hypo and takes less insulin. However the infection has increased his stress hormone levels so he really needs more, not less, and is admitted soon afterwards in hyperglycaemic coma. This is such a common mistake that all people on insulin need to be given clear 'sick day rules' (see Table 5.4).

The harmful effects of insulin deficiency have been explained on page 7 and in Fig. 1.4. In brief, glucose accumulates in the blood, spills over into the urine and draws out salt, water and potassium. The blood becomes increasingly concentrated and the tissues dehydrated (*hyperosmolar*), ultimately causing drowsiness or loss of consciousness (*coma*). Hyperglycaemia and ketosis cause vomiting and further fluid loss. More than anything else it is the onset of vomiting which makes the difference between a mild upset of diabetic control that the patient can treat himself and full-blown hyperglycaemic coma. One word of caution; the term 'coma' is potentially misleading because some patients remain fully conscious despite ketosis and hyperglycaemia. Hyperglycaemic coma presents differing proportions of hyperglycaemia, dehydration, acidosis and impaired consciousness in different patients.

Who can develop hyperglycaemic coma?

In theory, anyone with diabetes is at risk although the chances become smaller the later in life diabetes is diagnosed. Hyperglycaemic coma is commonest in adolescents and young adults and these are also the people most likely to have repeated episodes (like Susan, Case History 4.1). It is also easiest to *recognise* hyperglycaemic coma in younger people; in the elderly, particularly if they are not known to be diabetic, it is often overlooked until they are severely ill.

Precipitating causes

Infections and other illnesses (flu, gastroenteritis, pneumonia, urinary tract infections, heart attacks and strokes), mistakes with insulin doses and newly presenting diabetes are each responsible for about a quarter of cases and in a quarter no cause is found. Every patient admitted with hyperglycaemic coma must be examined carefully and have a chest X-ray, blood and urine culture and, after the age of 30, an e.c.g. to exclude a 'silent' heart attack (see page 171). If no cause is found, this must be recorded honestly in the notes. Girls like Susan have usually had half a dozen episodes of hyperglycaemic coma attributed to 'probable virus infections' before the real cause is discovered.

The clinical picture of hyperglycaemic coma

The history varies between a few hours, days or weeks. Older patients with non-insulin-dependent diabetes, in particular, may slip into hyperglycaemic coma so slowly that the diagnosis is missed and their forgetfulness, drowsiness and incontinence are put down to 'old age'. The symptoms of severe hyperglycaemia are thirst, polyuria, nocturia, weakness, a poor appetite, nausea and vomiting. Sometimes the symptoms of a precipitating illness like a heart attack may predominate. Severe abdominal pain which mimics a perforated ulcer can be caused by ketoacidosis, and it is not unheard of for such patients to spend 24 h on a surgical ward or even to have a laparotomy before hyperglycaemic coma is diagnosed.

The typical picture of hyperglycaemic coma is a pale, drowsy, cold patient with sunken eyes, a rapid thready pulse and a low blood pressure. Deep sighing respiration and a smell of ketones on the breath (reminiscent of pear drops) are signs of ketosis. *This is a medical emergency which needs immediate treatment.*

Treatment of hyperglycaemic coma

The doctor takes a quick history from the patient or his family, carries out an examination to assess the degree of dehydration and looks for signs of a precipitating illness. The diagnosis is confirmed by a bedside blood glucose measurement and a urine test for ketones. Blood is sent urgently to the laboratory for plasma sodium, potassium, urea and glucose determinations and a drip is started. All this should be done within 20 min of arriving in casualty.

Treatment from now on can be considered under the headings of medical care (fluid, insulin and electrolyte therapy) and nursing care (general care of the drowsy or unconscious patient, care of drips, insulin pumps, nasogastric tubes and catheters, and observation of the patient's progress).

Medical management

The doctor's job is to judge the rate of fluid, electrolyte and insulin replacement to:

- Bring the blood pressure up quickly if the patient is shocked.
- Bring blood glucose down to about 10 mmol/l within 6–24 h (depending on how high it is to start with).
- Correct the deficit of sodium and potassium.
- Give back the 5 l or so of water which have been lost.

Fluid and electrolytes

A plasma expander (plasma protein fraction or a synthetic substitute) is the treatment for shock (systolic blood pressure below 100 mmHg). Thereafter, 0.9% saline is the usual intravenous fluid although 0.45% saline may be needed for hyperosmolar coma or sodium bicarbonate for severe acidosis. How quickly the fluid is given depends on the severity of dehydration and whether there is heart or kidney failure; particularly in the elderly, fluid may have to be given slowly and central venous pressure monitored to prevent heart failure. Normally 1000–1500 ml of saline are given in the first hour, and 500–1000 ml in each of the next 4 h. No potassium is added to the first 500 ml of saline, but 1 g potassium chloride (KCl) is added to each 500 ml thereafter depending on the plasma potassium level.

Insulin

Insulin is best given intravenously by syringe pump starting at a rate of 6 units/h, increased if necessary. When the blood glucose is down to 10–15 mmol/l, 5% dextrose is added to the intravenous fluid regimen and the insulin infusion rate adjusted to maintain blood sugar at this level (using a sliding scale, see also Table 5.9, p. 103).

Precipitating causes, complications and progress

The doctor has to keep a watch for signs of a precipitating illness even if none is apparent when he first examines the patient. Antibiotics may need to be given to the severely ill because there is no time to wait for the results of cultures. Severely dehydrated patients, particularly the elderly, are often anticoagulated with heparin because there is a high risk of arterial thrombosis. Fluid, potassium and insulin requirements cannot be predicted accurately at the outset, so close clinical observation and frequent blood glucose and potassium measurements are the cornerstones of good care.

Nursing care

Care of the airway

Drowsiness is usual and severely ill patients may be deeply comatose so protection of the airway is the first priority. Remember that vomiting is a symptom of ketosis and may not start until the patient begins to regain consciousness. A nasogastric tube should always be inserted if he is any more than slightly drowsy because the ketoacidotic patient often has a dilated stomach (*gastric stasis*) and may vomit profusely and aspirate the contents.

Observations

Blood pressure and pulse should be monitored at least hourly because hypotension and tachycardia are signs of dehydration. It is common for patients in hyperglycaemic coma to be hypothermic, sometimes profoundly so, in which case the temperature should be monitored with a low reading thermometer. Frequent measurement is important because patients with a normal or low temperature on admission may become pyrexial soon afterwards if they have an underlying infection. This must be recognised promptly and reported to the doctor. If a reflectance meter is available, blood glucose monitoring is another important nursing duty; at first the level may be off the top of the scale of the meter but the nurse must recognise when the blood glucose is approaching the target of 10 mmol/l and maintain it at this level with a sliding scale.

Oral fluids, urine output and catheters

No matter how thirsty he is, the patient should not drink more than sips of water because of the risk of vomiting; he/she can suck ice cubes to moisten his/her mouth. The urine output should be monitored and renal failure suspected if it fails to increase after adequate rehydration; this should prompt caution with fluid replacement. A catheter should be avoided if the patient is well enough to use a bottle or bedpan (because of the risk of ascending infection) but is necessary if he/she is in renal failure, unconscious, severely ill or goes into retention.

Drips and pumps

It is a truism to say that drips should run to time; however, it is the nurse's responsibility to ensure that the patient is rapidly resuscitated in the early stages of treatment. Once the blood glucose has been controlled and the sliding scale is being used, the rate of dextrose infusion has to be kept absolutely constant. The nurses on a diabetes ward should, ideally, have ready access to syringe pumps and understand them well because intravenous insulin infusions are the best way of managing diabetes during surgery, labour and intercurrent illness as well as hyperglycaemic coma.

DIABETES AND EXERCISE

Case History 4.2

Darren, an energetic 16-year-old, has just moved up to the sixth form at school. Two of his friends are planning to run a half-marathon; Darren would like to train with them and give his sponsorship money to the British Diabetic Association. His friends are not keen on the idea because they do not believe that someone with diabetes could stand the training. This makes him all the more determined to run and he seeks advice from the diabetic clinic.

Can people with diabetes take part in sports?

An insulin-dependent diabetic can take part in almost any sport. Hang-gliding, parachute jumping and subaqua diving are discouraged, not because diabetes makes them impossible but because hypoglycaemia in midair or underwater is disastrous. Marathon running (Fig. 4.1) and other competitive sports require careful preparation but diabetics have made successful professionals in football, tennis and cricket. To understand what preparation is required, consider how exercise affects diabetes and vice versa.

How does exercise affect diabetes?

Exercise burns up carbohydrate, speeds insulin absorption by increasing blood flow to injection sites and, after prolonged training, reduces insulin requirements by making the body more sensitive to insulin. All will tend to lower blood glucose so hypoglycaemia is the main effect of exercise; this may occur not just during exercise but up to several hours afterwards when the carbohydrate stores in the liver and muscle are being replenished.

How does diabetes affect exercise?

Ideally, it should have no effect at all. Hypoglycaemia can wreck sporting performance, as can hyperglycaemia. The athlete has to walk a tightrope between these two extremes by matching insulin doses and diet carefully before and during exercise. Finally, misguided and overprotective parents and friends may undermine the person's confidence in his/her sporting ability.

What benefits does exercise have for the person with diabetes?

Some benefits are the same as for non-diabetics; exercise tends to lower blood lipid concentrations and blood pressure and generally 'tone up' the system. Other benefits are unique to diabetes; exercise may lower blood glucose and insulin requirements. Obesity is a problem for many diabetics and regular exercise is one solution. All these changes are good for diabetics because they tend to protect against heart disease.

How should an insulin-dependent diabetic prepare for exercise?

First, he must build up his pattern of exercise gradually and work out by trial and error how to strike the balance between exercise, diet and insulin doses. Darren might, for example, start by running for 20 min before his evening meal 3 nights a week, increasing by 10 min each week. His evening insulin injection could be delayed until after the run and he would probably need 30 g of rapidly available carbohydrate (dextrose tablets, chocolate or a sugary drink) beforehand. He should carry glucose tablets with him, perhaps in a pocket specially sewn into his running shorts. It is no bad thing for him to have company while he is gettting into training in case he misjudges. With practice, he may well be able to return from his training with a normal blood glucose. His morning and evening insulin doses may be able to come down by 8 units with better overall control. He must notify the organisers of the marathon that he has diabetes and carry with him his diabetic identification card and plenty of glucose tablets. More general advice is given in Table 4.2 and discussed below.

If exercise is to be taken soon after an insulin injection, the dose

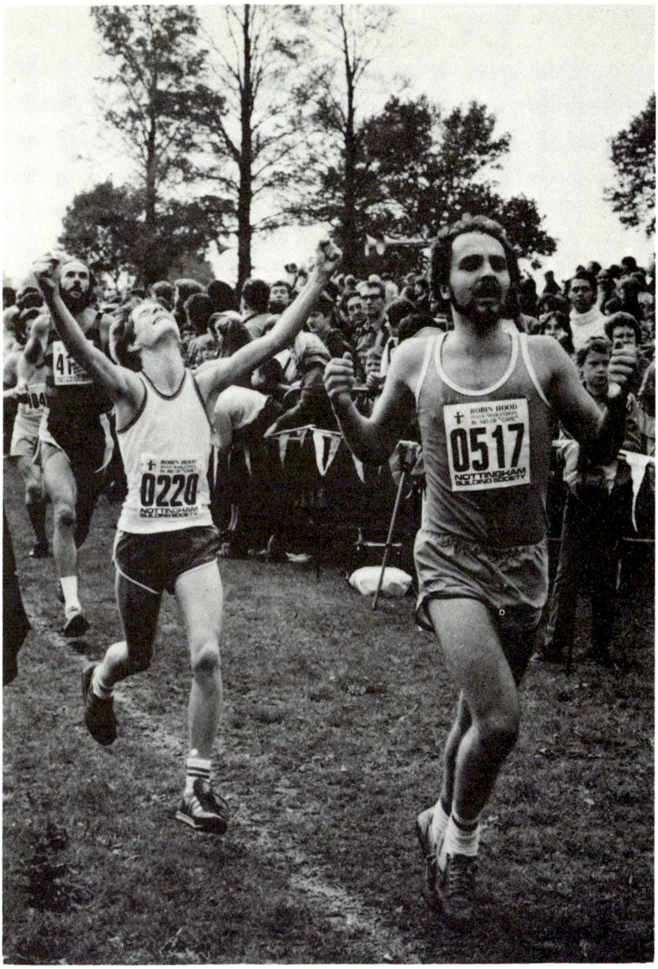

Fig. 4.1 Running the Nottingham marathon.

of short-acting insulin can be reduced by 4–6 units. Injecting insulin into the abdomen rather than the thigh or arm reduces the risk of hypoglycaemia because it is less affected by increased blood flow during exercise. While the choice between taking extra carbohydrate or reducing the dose of insulin is usually a matter of habit or convenience, it makes more sense for someone who is trying to lose weight to cut down their insulin dose. Whichever method is chosen, the best results are achieved with the help of blood tests to

Table 4.2 How to prevent hypoglycaemia during exercise

If you will be exercising soon after an injection
Cut down the dose of short-acting insulin by 4–6 units
At other times
Take 20–30 g of extra carbohydrate as dextrose tablets, chocolate or a sugary drink immediately beforehand
Do a blood test immediately before, after and (if feasible) during sports to check that your predictions were accurate; find out by trial and error how to strike the right balance
Always carry glucose tablets with you

measure the effect on blood glucose. A test immediately before a game of football, during the interval and afterwards will quickly teach the sportsman how to keep himself in peak form. Dextrose tablets in a pocket will safeguard against severe hypoglycaemia during exercise and a meal or snack afterwards helps to protect against 'late hypoglycaemia'.

GROUP EDUCATION OF THE INSULIN-DEPENDENT DIABETIC

Case History 4.3

Karen is now 18. She has wanted to be a nurse for as long as she can remember but becoming diabetic at the age of 10 gave her extra incentive. Imagine her disappointment when the local school of nursing turned her down because she was on insulin. After several more disappointments, she has been given a place by a nursing school with a more enlightened attitude. However, she has always depended on her rather overprotective mother to prepare suitable meals and advise about her insulin; the start of her training is the first time she has been away from home and taken complete responsibility for her diabetes.

She has taken one injection of short-acting and long-acting insulin a day ever since diagnosis and rarely changes the dose because she has found that any attempt to get her urine sugar-free causes hypos in the afternoon or during the night. Now she is at the end of her introductory block and about to start shift work and worried sick about how she will manage.

The watershed between dependence and independence

Karen has been ill-prepared to leave home: her doctor has left her on an unsuitable insulin regimen with a second-rate method of monitoring and made no attempt to find out how much or little she knows about diabetes. Her parents have not encouraged her to take responsibility for her own care. Leaving home can be difficult enough without all these extra problems. The insulin regimen and monitoring can quickly be changed although building up her self-confidence will take longer.

Twice-daily injections of short-acting and medium-acting insulin will give more predictable control throughout the 24 h and greater flexibility for her changes of shift. It is worth taking this opportunity to check her technique of drawing up and injecting insulin. Monitoring blood rather than urine glucose gives more accurate information (see page 26) and, once she has seen the benefits, she is likely to accept the extra discomfort readily.

It might be tempting to stop here and think that the problem is solved but there is a danger that she will become as dependent on the nurse and doctor as she was on her mother. She must learn to be her own manager and use the diabetes team for support and advice. This is a time when group education has a lot to offer. Learning more about diabetes, knowing that others have the same problems and seeing how they cope with them should help encourage Karen's self-reliance.

Diabetes education: in or out of clinic?

A diabetic clinic is the worst possible place to teach because there is pressure of time; ill patients inevitably take priority and infrequent attenders coming for a check-up expect a thorough examination. Most 'problem-solving' and 'screening' has to be done one-to-one but, apart from teaching insulin-dependent diabetics in the first weeks after diagnosis (see Chapter 5), most teaching is best done in groups and *all* teaching is best away from the hurly-burly of the clinic.

Organising groups for insulin-dependent diabetic patients

The general pros and cons of group education are discussed in Chapter 7. This section describes specifically the approach to re-educating young insulin-dependent diabetics. Groups work best if

Table 4.3 Outline of a series of group education sessions for insulin-dependent diabetic patients

Week 1	*Week 2*	*Week 3*	*Week 4*
Short quiz to find out how much the participants know	Quiz using food models to calculate the carbohydrate content of meals	Small groups to discuss fears about complications	Participants report back on their previous week's task
Video showing a humorous interview with a diabetic celebrity	Split up into small groups to create an imaginative and varied menu from one member's carbohydrate distribution	Small groups report back to the whole group	How to cope with insulin during illness
Principles of diet and the effect of refined carbohydrate on blood glucose	Food tasting when participants can taste various high fibre recipes	Discussion about large vessel disease and the evils of smoking	Contraception and pregnancy
Each group member is asked to record his carbohydrate intake over a 3 day period during the next week to see how constant it is	Discussion of hypoglycaemia and the use of glucagon	How different insulins act and how to alter insulin doses	Holidays and travel
		Other ways of giving insulin such as pens and pumps	Driving and insurance
		Each participant has the task of altering their insulin in response to a change of routine during the coming week	British Diabetic Association and other patients support groups
			A 'lay adviser' joins the group to answer questions

the number of patients is around eight and the members are of roughly similar age; Karen is one of eight diabetic patients in their late teens and early 20s. There are four sessions to allow enough time to cover the ground without them becoming a chore, and the group meets weekly to maintain the impetus. All participants are encouraged to bring their nearest and dearest with them so they have moral support and someone to ask if they forget what was discussed. The groups are held during the evening so as not to interfere with work or college. The atmosphere is relaxed and informal and first names are used. The team who run the group should consist at least of a nurse, doctor and dietitian and all should, ideally, attend all four sessions. Table 4.3 outlines suggestions for the content of the sessions.

Content of group education sessions for insulin-dependent diabetics

Week 1

Diet may give more trouble to people with diabetes than any other aspect of their care. Taking Lucozade and showing how quickly it increases blood sugar brings home the effect of refined carbohydrate on diabetic control. It also illustrates that most people cannot tell whether their blood glucose level is 8 or 18 mmol/l by the way they feel; hence the need to do blood glucose tests. This session also introduces the use of blood glucose meters.

Week 2

This is also largely devoted to diet. Participants are split into small groups and helped to become more familiar with the principles of carbohydrate distribution by planning menus for one another. The diabetes team have cooked dishes to illustrate what palatable meals can be prepared from high fibre foods. Examples are:

- Lasagne made with wholemeal pasta
- Bean paella
- Wholemeal banana bread

Many other interesting ideas can be found in *The Diabetics Diet Book* (see p. 110).

This session finishes with a discussion of the symptoms, causes and prevention of hypoglycaemia. The use of glucagon is described and, above all else, the participants are reassessed that hypoglycaemia rarely causes serious harm, even if it occurs during sleep.

Week 3

Most diabetic patients know or have heard of a diabetic who has lost a limb or gone blind. Professionals do not like to discuss such a distasteful subject with their patients but the best way of tackling it is to take a positive approach and emphasise how these disasters can be avoided. By this stage, the participants know one another well enough to voice their fears and group dynamics can encourage mutual support and reassurance. It must be clearly spelt out that smoking magnifies the risks of heart disease and gangrene in people with diabetes.

Again, the group are encouraged to learn by participation; in the last part of this session, each is given the task of adjusting their insulin and diet at least once during the forthcoming week to maintain as good control as possible during a departure from their normal routine (a late meal after a concert, for example).

Week 4

Each participant reports back on the task he was set a week ago and the whole group discusses their experiences. The topic of pregnancy is raised; diabetic girls are told of the need for excellent control even before conception and advised to contact their doctor in good time if they are contemplating pregnancy. Information is given about motor insurance, travel and life assurance (Table 4.4). Finally, a 'lay adviser' attends for the last half-hour of the session. This is a 'well-adjusted' person with long-standing insulin-dependent diabetes who can answer questions from a patient's point of view.

Apart from boosting her confidence and equipping her to deal with the practicalities, Karen now knows her doctor, nurse and dietitian as friends and will have no hesitation about approaching them for advice. She may now find it easier to face up to complications, something of which she will be constantly reminded during her nursing career. Her new knowledge and future experience should give her a special understanding of the needs of other diabetic patients.

Table 4.4 Diabetes and insurance

Life insurance	Policies taken out before diagnosis remain valid; it should be possible to take out a new policy after diagnosis, depending on medical reports, but the premium will probably be high
Travel	Medical insurance is a must because bills can be exorbitant, particularly in the United States; diabetes must be declared on the application form or the insurance may be invalidated
Driving	Whether on diet alone, tablets or insulin, diabetes must be notified to the insurer; again, the premium may be high. The British Diabetic Association can recommend companies which are sympathetic to the diabetic

Shift work

Karen's new insulin regimen provides reasonable flexibility for shift work. The doses of medium-acting insulin before breakfast and the evening meal can be left unchanged, whatever the time, and the dose of short-acting insulin varied depending on what she eats. Frequent blood tests, at least in the early stages, help to guide these adjustments. As a nurse, she can call in to the ward clinical room to do a test whenever she needs to, though others (particularly manual workers) may find this impossible. A multiple injection regimen (see page 132) is more flexible still for people working irregular hours; this is discussed on page 131.

HYPOGLYCAEMIA, ALCOHOL AND DIABETES

Hypoglycaemia occurs when the blood glucose falls below 2.5 mmol/l. Apart from some rare endocrine diseases such as insulin-secreting tumours of the pancreas, it is always caused by insulin or sulphonylureas (glibenclamide, chlorpropamide or tolbutamide). It has two main effects: (1) the brain is deprived of glucose, its only fuel; and (2) the body attempts to counteract this by pouring out the 'stress hormones' (mainly adrenaline, noradrenaline and glucagon) which have actions opposite to those of insulin.

Symptoms of hypoglycaemia

These are summarised in Table 4.5. An 'adrenaline surge' causes the characteristic warning symptoms of trembling, sweating and palpitations. Shortage of glucose in the brain causes faintness, lightheadedness, tingling in the fingers, drowsiness, confusion or aggressive behaviour and, ultimately, unconsciousness and fits. Any or all of these symptoms may occur in a hypoglycaemic reaction (otherwise known as a *hypo*, *insulin reaction*, *reaction* or *insulin shock*). Different people get different combinations of symptoms, although they may be remarkably consistent within the same individual. Some may become sweaty and shaky long before their judgement is seriously impaired, giving them plenty of time to recognise what is wrong and take sugar. For others who are less fortunate, drowsiness or aggressive behaviour is the first sign and their judgement is already too badly affected to recognise what is wrong and take sugar. Wives and husbands can often pick up the early signs of hypoglycaemia before their partner. After having diabetes for many years, the warning signs may change or disappear completely, leaving the diabetic vulnerable to recurrent hypoglycaemia.

Any odd behaviour in an insulin-dependent diabetic should be regarded as hypoglycaemia until proved otherwise. If there is doubt, the proof is whether or not they respond to sugar; adequate carbohydrate should correct the symptoms in less than half an hour. Here are circumstances in which a hypo might happen:

Table 4.5 Symptoms and signs of hypoglycaemia

Things the patient may notice	*Things other people may notice*	*Cause*
Faintness Hunger Blurred vision Headache	Irritability Personality change Glazed look in the eyes	Nervous system deprived of glucose
Palpitations Excessive sweating Trembling	Pallor	Adrenaline secretion

Case History 4.4

Steven, aged 19 and working as a lorry driver for a builders' merchant, goes drinking with his mates every Friday and Saturday. Friday is a friend's birthday and, knowing that he will be drinking more than usual, he takes his normal dose of insulin at 6 pm but skips his meal so that he can substitute pints of beer for his usual carbohydrate exchanges. Shortly before closing time, his speech becomes slurred and then he becomes unusually quiet. Not knowing that he is diabetic, his mates assume that he has had too much to drink and ignore him. The next thing they know, he is on the floor. They cannot rouse him so the landlord of the pub calls an ambulance. A fingerprick blood test in casualty registers a blood glucose level of only 1 mmol/l.

How common is severe hypoglycaemia?

If defined as an incident where the person cannot recognise or control themselves, and which requires treatment with glucagon or glucose (see below), approximately one-third of people treated with insulin will have such an episode during their diabetic lifetimes, and one in ten will have at least one per year. Occasional people never experience a hypo, perhaps because they are so badly controlled that their blood glucose is never below 10 mmol/l. Remember that hypoglycaemia, though associated in most peoples' minds just with insulin, is also caused by oral hypoglycaemics (see page 181) and can easily be overlooked in the elderly.

What causes hypoglycaemia?

The common causes are delayed or missed meals, strenuous exercise, too high insulin doses and alcohol (see below, page 82). In some people, hypos are unpredictable, while others have them only if they depart from their normal routine.

What effects does it have?

Many diabetic patients' worst unspoken fear is that they will die during a hypo while asleep. In practice, hypoglycaemia almost never kills unless the patient is parachute jumping or driving a car at the time. However, serious brain damage can be caused by severe hypoglycaemia lasting for more than 8 h but this is usually caused by attempted suicide (or murder!). Hypoglycaemia in the elderly may masquerade as a stroke or, if the person is living alone and profoundly hypoglycaemic for many hours, may even *cause* a stroke. In general, hypoglycaemia does not have permanent physical consequences although it can disrupt social or professional life and seriously undermine self-confidence.

Treatment

Most hypos are treated by the patient; 20–30 g of refined carbohydrate taken as sugar lumps, dextrose tablets, Lucozade, chocolate or milk and biscuits will usually cure the symptoms within 5 min. If the hypo gets to the point where the person will not or cannot swallow, it is sometimes possible to bring them round by smearing a sticky glucose solution (Hypostop) on their tongues or in their cheeks. If all else fails, glucagon or intravenous glucose is needed. However, intravenous glucose has two great disadvantages: the injection requires skill plus a second pair of hands to keep the patient still; the sticky glucose solution may damage veins which will be needed in the future. Glucagon, a hormone normally produced by the pancreas, releases glucose from the liver and can be given by anyone who has been shown how to use the kit. Practical details of glucagon administration are shown in Appendix 6.

How to teach patients about hypoglycaemia and its prevention

Many lay people are aware that diabetics can suddenly lose consciousness, and this may be one of the greatest fears in the minds of a patient and his family at the start of insulin treatment. Discussing the symptoms and ways of preventing hypoglycaemia is an early priority of education. Often talking to another person with diabetes helps allay anxiety. It is important to stress that occasional mild hypos are not a bad thing and indicate that blood glucose is close to normal at least some of the time. Frequent or severe hypoglycaemia is a different matter and may require adjustments in the diet or insulin dose; it is best to keep a record and report hypos at clinic visits. When a doctor asks 'how many hypos have you had?', he is interested in minor symptoms as well as loss of consciousness.

Table 4.6 Some important points for avoiding hypoglycaemic comas (hypos)

• Do not miss meals or snacks and eat them punctually
• Carry enough glucose at all times—once the symptoms of hypoglycaemia come on, you cannot wait until you get home or reach the next shop
• Take special precautions when driving or during exercise; remember that 'exercise' includes pushing the car in snow, mowing the lawn, decorating the house and making love!
• Make sure that your workmates or lovers know that you are diabetic, know the symptoms of hypos and what to do about them

Table 4.6 summarises some important points about preventing hypos.

Special situations

Precautions against hypoglycaemia during exercise are covered on page 72, and driving in Chapter 6.

Nocturnal hypoglycaemia

This deserves special mention because it may be particularly dreaded by some and not recognised by others. 'How will I know if I have a hypo during sleep?' is a question often asked. Husbands or wives are often disturbed by unusual restlessness or profuse sweating. Sometimes the diabetic may wake with a splitting headache or feel 'hungover' for no apparent reason. Rarely, hypoglycaemia causes fits during the night.

It is usually unhelpful to measure blood glucose the next morning because by then it will have risen as the previous night's injection 'runs out'. The only certain way to detect hypos during sleep is for the patient or spouse to set the alarm clock for 3 am and do a blood test. This may need to be done several nights running to rule out hypoglycaemia.

Nocturnal hypos can be prevented in several ways: by taking a larger bedtime snack; by reducing the evening medium-acting insulin; or by shifting the evening injection of medium-acting insulin from before the evening meal to before bed (so that its peak action is 6 or 7 pm rather than 3 am; see page 19).

Table 4.7 Advice about drinking alcohol for patients on insulin

- The symptoms of hypoglycaemia may be like drunkenness—unsteadiness on the feet, slurred speech and aggressive behaviour. If you have had a drink, a hypo may not be recognised. Carry identification and warn your friends that you are diabetic
- Do not miss out carbohydrate if you plan to drink
- Alcoholic drinks containing little carbohydrate (dry wine, spirits, low calorie beers) are most suitable. If you have carbohydrate-containing alcoholic drinks, do not count them into your allowance
- Alcohol, like most things, is best taken in moderation

The effect of alcohol on blood glucose

At least Steven (Case History 4.4) tried to allow for the extra carbohydrate in his beer but he made several mistakes that spoilt his evening out. He took his normal insulin but left out his evening meal. The delay before taking carobohydrate could in itself have caused him to have a hypo but he ran up against another problem; he took an equivalent amount of carobohydrate in the form of beer but did not realise that alcohol tends to lower blood glucose (by preventing the liver from releasing glucose) despite the carbohydrate in it, and the net result was disastrous. His other big mistake was not to tell his friends that he was diabetic. Had they known, they might have recognised the signs of hypoglycaemia and persuaded him to eat something before it was too late. Of course, Steven's social life must not be spoilt by diabetes but he cannot achieve this just by turning his back on it. The advice he needs to keep himself out of trouble in future is summarised in Table 4.7.

Further reading

Barker P. (1981) *Basic Family Therapy*. London: Granada Publishing. An introduction to the techniques of family therapy.

Farquhar J. (1982) *Diabetes in your Teens. Patient Handbook Series.* Edinburgh: Churchill Livingstone. For adolescent diabetic patients.

Tattersall R. B., Lowe J. (1981) Diabetes in adolescence. *Diabetologia*; 20: 517–523.

5/

Diabetes in young adult life

INTRODUCTION

Almost all young diabetic adults are insulin-dependent; some have had diabetes since childhood or adolescence but others develop it in early adult life. Rarely, non-insulin-dependent diabetes may present in young adults, particularly if they are very fat or have a strong family history of diabetes. This chapter discusses some typical aspects of insulin-dependent diabetes in this age group.

- *David develops insulin-dependent diabetes at the age of 25. Does he need to be admitted to hospital, how should he start insulin treatment and what else does he need to be taught?*
- *Judith is on insulin and starts to put on weight. Is her insulin treatment to blame and how should she set about slimming?*
- *Lesley wants to start a family. What are the problems of diabetic pregnancy and how is she looked after during pregnancy and labour?*
- *Jane develops an unsightly red rash on her legs, a condition called 'necrobiosis'. How common is this in people with diabetes and what treatment is there?*

NEW DIABETES IN A YOUNG ADULT

A sudden onset of weight loss and other typical symptoms of diabetes in a young person strongly suggest insulin-dependent diabetes (see pages 11–13). A raised blood sugar (usually over 15 mmol/l) and ketones in the urine clinch the diagnosis.

Case History 5.1

David is 25, married and works as an electrician. Just before his summer holiday he begins to feel completely exhausted, and finds that everything is a big effort. He and his wife Sally put this down to overwork but he feels no better on holiday and starts drinking pints of lemonade. At first they blame the hot weather, but realise something is really wrong when he starts to lose weight and his clothes do not fit. On their return home they go to their general practitioner who finds glucose in David's urine. The doctor telephones the hospital immediately and David is seen in the diabetic clinic that afternoon.

David would inevitably have gone into ketoacidosis within days or weeks without insulin and this delay could have been fatal. The consultant has to decide whether he should start insulin in hospital or at home.

Starting insulin as an adult: hospital or home?

If a diabetes liaison sister is available to see patients at home, few adults who are well enough to come to clinic need admission. Moderate or severe dehydration and ketosis are the most usual reasons; others are summarised in Table 5.1. Young children are more often admitted to start insulin while their parents come to terms with diabetes (see Case History 3.1), but even the importance of this is questioned.

The practicalities of the first injection

The thought of having to inject yourself with insulin each day for the rest of your life is a shock which can be underestimated by pro-

Table 5.1 Reasons for admitting a newly diagnosed insulin-dependent diabetic adult to hospital

- Repeated vomiting or dehydration
- Moderate or severe ketosis
- Serious associated diseases (for example, chest infection)
- Poor home support or difficulty managing injections

Table 5.2 Priorities for the first day of insulin treatment

- A brief explanation of diabetes and the action of insulin
- How to draw up and give an insulin injection
  go slowly and keep it simple
  demonstrate the injection on yourself first
  teach how to inject before drawing up
- Injection sites
- Times and doses of injections
- How to store insulin and syringes
- How to recognise hypoglycaemia and what to do about it
- A day and night telephone number for problems, queries and reassurance

fessionals familiar with syringes and needles. David and Sally will be extremely worried, though relieved to hear that he does not have to be admitted to hospital. Remember that they will absorb little of what they are told in this frame of mind so it has to be kept simple. The priorities are summarised in Table 5.2.

Keep it simple and informal

The explanation of diabetes should be as simple as possible. Giving the first injection is a big hurdle which should not be delayed; the sooner it is done, the sooner David can relax and absorb what he is told. Where this is done is important. Most people find it least stressful at home but even hospital rooms can be made informal with easy chairs, pictures and plants. It must be somewhere private; if the telephone rings constantly and people are knocking at the door, neither patient nor teacher can concentrate. Technical details of drawing up and giving an insulin injection are illustrated in Appendices 1 to 3, but the most important points are emphasised here.

Demonstrate on yourself first

Before asking David to give his own injection, the nurse should show him how to do it by injecting herself with an empty syringe. This may sound dreadful but proves that injections do not really hurt and gives tremendous confidence. If the nurse does not have the courage to do it, how can David be expected to?

Sticking the needle in

Immediately after demonstrating on herself, she should encourage David to give his own injection. Drawing up insulin is quite complicated; if this is explained before he has 'stuck in the needle' he will be so apprehensive that he will not absorb a word of the explanation. It is immensely rewarding to hear the sigh of relief after a successful first injection. To a person who has just been diagnosed diabetic, it is the biggest step in the world and deserves praise.

Step by step

The whole process of drawing up and injecting insulin should then be explained and practised in short steps (see Appendix 1). This has to be taken slowly and repeated as often as necessary until David has mastered the technique and gained self-confidence.

How much insulin, how often and when?

Above all, the insulin regimen should be kept simple. It is good practice to start with *two* injections a day because good control can rarely be achieved in the long run on a single injection. Mixing short-acting and medium-acting insulin is a complication which should be avoided at the start. No formula can predict the right insulin dose so it is sensible to begin with a small dose and build up. For example, 10 units of intermediate-acting insulin morning and evening are easy to draw up, do not involve mixing insulins and are unlikely to cause hypoglycaemia, which would quickly destroy David's self-confidence. The injections are given 20–30 min before both breakfast and evening meal. The dose can be increased and short-acting insulin added once David has mastered injections.

Injection sites and equipment

Injecting insulin and swabbing the skin

Insulin can be injected wherever there is fat; the usual sites are shown in Fig. 5.1. It is more important to encourage people to vary their injection sites systematically than to use particular sites at particular times. Repeated injections in one spot make the tissue below the skin hard and lumpy and the insulin absorption erratic;

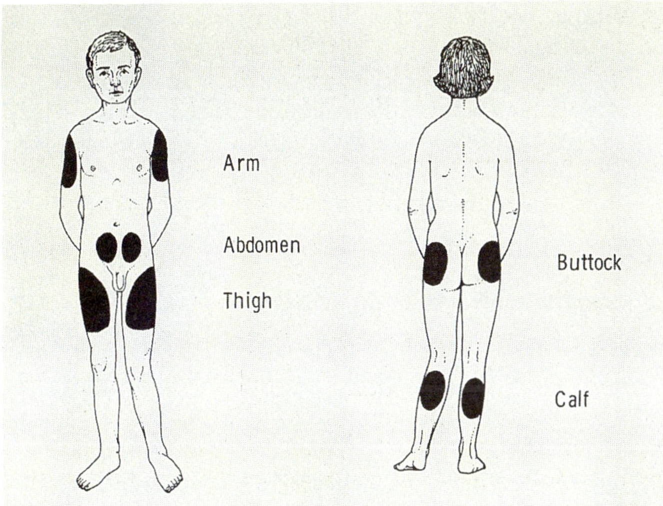

Fig. 5.1 Usual sites for insulin injections. From Tattersall (1986), reproduced with permission.

this is called *lipohypertrophy* (see p. 89). A simple routine is to inject the abdomen in the morning and the thigh or buttock in the evening. 'Is it necessary to swab the skin?' is a frequent question. Provided it is clean, there is no need to swab it with spirit before injections. Apart from complicating the ritual, spirit toughens the skin and, if not allowed to dry, makes the injections sting.

Storing insulin

The current bottle of insulin can be kept at room temperature, away from radiators and direct sunlight. Insulin loses only 10% of its potency if left at room temperature for a year, so short periods out of the fridge do no harm. Spare bottles should be kept in the fridge, not the freezer.

Types of syringes

Plastic syringes are convenient, have fine sharp needles and are now prescribable under the NHS. Although the manufacturers specify that they should only be used once, it is quite safe to reuse them until the needle is blunt, the markings on the barrel wear off or the plunger begins to stick. Preservatives in the insulin help to keep the syringe sterile, so it is only necessary to replace the cap over the needle and store the syringe in a clean place. A glass syringe with detachable needles and a plastic carrying case can also be prescribed but most people find plastic syringes much more convenient.

Introducing the subject of hypoglycaemia

Little need be said about hypoglyaemia at this stage because it is uncommon within the first few days of treatment unless an unnecessarily large dose of insulin has been prescribed. In the past, many doctors and nurses felt that it was important to induce a hypo deliberately so that patients would learn the symptoms, but this is best avoided because it may be very threatening to someone who has just started insulin, and the symptoms are quite easy to recognise. It is sufficient to say that: 'insulin can cause the blood sugar to drop too low and the symptoms to look out for are a headache, shaking, excessive hunger, or weakness. Typically these occur after activity or when a meal is due. Dextrose tablets, sugar lumps or sweets should be carried at *all* times (particularly if driving) and taken immediately if these symptoms develop'. (See Case History 4.4, page 78.)

What else needs to be taught on the first day?

All that is important is that David is able to give injections confidently and knows not to miss them even if he does not feel like eating. He should eat regular meals to prevent hypoglycaemia and cut out sugar, but more detailed dietary advice would be confusing at this stage. Urine or blood testing is another complication to be avoided until he has mastered drawing up and injecting insulin. A booklet giving a simple description of diabetes and its treatment is helpful; several excellent ones are available (see page 110). Finally, David and Sally need both nurse's and doctor's telephone numbers to ring if they have problems. This gives confidence and is rarely abused. A telephone call from the nurse the next day and a home visit soon afterwards will give extra support during these difficult early days.

PROBLEMS AT INJECTION SITES

Lipoatrophy

As its name indicates, this is wasting of fat which usually occurs at the site of repeated injections and causes unsightly hollows (Fig. 5.2a). It is most commonly (though not exclusively) caused by impure beef insulins and is thought to be a type of local allergic reaction. With the increasing use of pork and human insulins, it is becoming less common. While lipoatrophy is disfiguring, it is harmless and can usually be improved by changing the patient to purified pork or human insulin and injecting it directly into the hollows.

Lipohypertrophy

A lump over the thigh, abdomen or arm usually indicates that the patient is giving all his injections in the same spot, perhaps because he has discovered that this makes them painless. Apart from being unattractive, lipohypertrophy may cause erratic insulin absorption and unstable control. It can occur with any type of insulin and the only treatment is to vary the injection sites (Fig 5.2b).

Local allergy to insulin

Rarely, some patients develop a red, itchy 'nettle-rash' in the first 2–3 weeks of insulin therapy. It will usually subside on its own within weeks but a change of insulin should be considered if it persists.

Injection site abscesses

Though relatively rare, the risk of an abscess has traditionally been given as the reason for sterilising syringes and swabbing the skin with spirit before injecting. In practice, these measures do not prevent abscesses and have been abandoned. Once an abscess is established, surgical drainage is usually necessary.

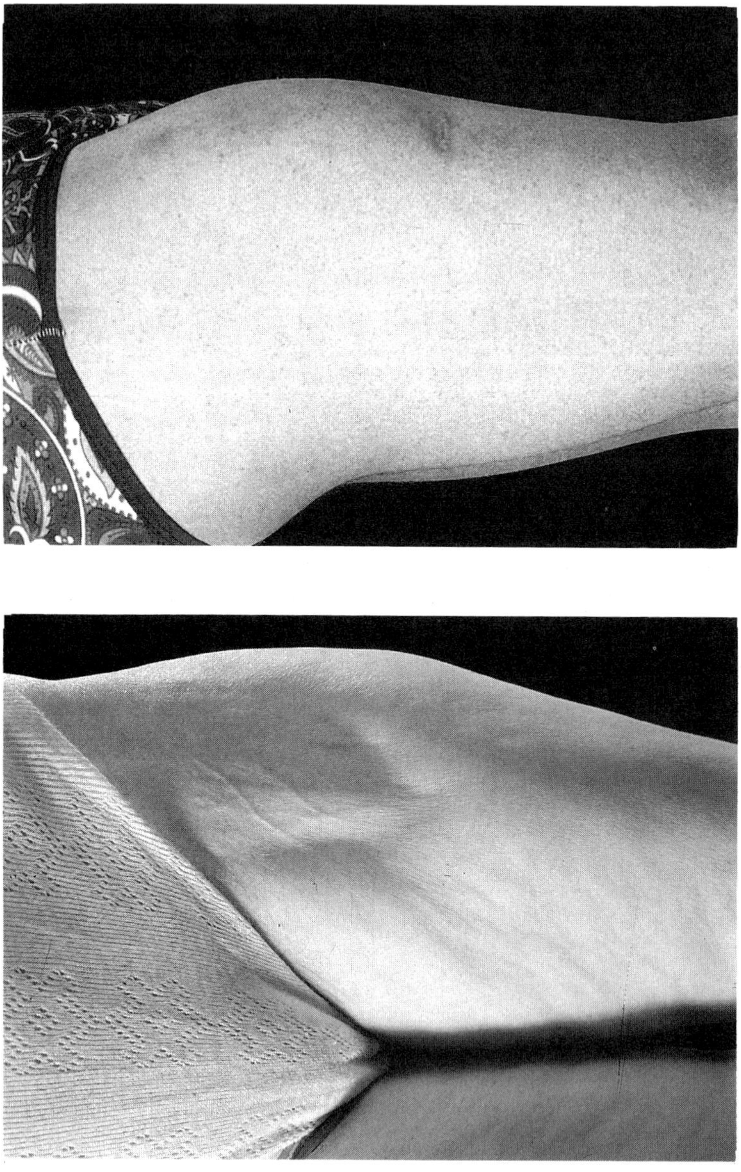

Fig. 5.2 (a) An example of lipoatrophy. (b) An example of lipohypertrophy.

EDUCATION OF THE RECENTLY DIAGNOSED INSULIN-INDEPENDENT DIABETIC

Diabetes, of all chronic diseases, is the one where it is most important for the patient to 'be his own doctor'. David has taken the first step towards independence by giving his own injections but there is much more to learn; in particular, how to achieve a stable blood sugar by balancing what he eats against his insulin doses and exercise. Looking back on it afterwards, people usually say that the diagnosis of diabetes came as a terrible shock to them. To lose good health can strike as hard as the loss of a close friend and may take months to come to terms with. No two individuals are alike in the time it takes them to adjust. It is important to remember what David is going through and not to rush the process of teaching as much of what he is told will be completely foreign. On the other hand, once the excitement of starting insulin is over, it is easy for his teachers to forget details which are none the less important.

Monitoring, diet and exercise

In the early weeks, the fact that David regains weight and energy and stops feeling thirsty is a good indication that things are getting back to normal; however, he needs a more sensitive way of testing in the long run. The pros and cons of urine and blood testing have been discussed in Chapter 1. Most young adults have no difficulty pricking their fingers and, for them, blood testing is the obvious choice. If they are needle-shy it is wise not to introduce finger-pricking until they are established on insulin.

Most people with diabetes say that diet (and the carbohydrate exchange system in particular) is the aspect of their treatment which is most complicated and most interferes with their lives. Detailed dietary teaching should start when David and Sally have come to terms with the diagnosis and are ready to absorb a lot of new information. Both of them must be involved in planning his diet since it will affect the whole household. They will have to accept some changes, but unless their food preferences and normal routine are taken into consideration they may well end up ignoring all the advice they are given. The dietary principles for insulin-dependent diabetes are described on pages 93–4.

A young adult like David who is still underweight and has a big appetite may need at least 2500 calories per day; a 280 g (28 exchange) carbohydrate diet divided up into three meals and two

Table 5.3 Two sample menus providing identical carbohydrate distributions

	Exchanges	*Total carbohydrate exchanges*	*Exchanges*	
		Breakfast		
Two shredded wheat	2	3		Half grapefruit
1/3 pint milk	1			Egg, bacon and tomato
Cup of tea			3	Two medium slices wholemeal toast
				Marmalade
		Snack		
Two medium slices wholemeal bread; cheese and tomato filling	3	3	3	Wholemeal date scone
Cup of coffee				Coffee
		Lunch		
Four medium slices wholemeal bread; cheese and tomato filling	6	8	1	Bowl of cream of chicken soup
				Roast beef, peas, cauliflower, carrots
One packet cheese and onion crisps	1		2	Two roast potatoes
			2	Two Yorkshire puddings
Apple	1			
Cup of tea			3	Black forest gateau with cream
				Coffee
		Evening meal		
Roast chicken, gravy, carrots and brussel sprouts		10	5	Half a medium deep pan pizza
				Mixed salad
Two large jacket potatoes	6		2	Portion of garlic bread
			3	Banana split, ice cream
Apple pie	3			Coffee
Custard	1			
Coffee				
		Bedtime snack		
Two medium slices wholemeal toast	3	3	2	Two digestive biscuits
Cup of tea			1	Milky drink
		Milk for drinks during the day		
		1		
		Total daily carbohydrate		
		28		
		(1 exchange = 10 g carbohydrate)		

snacks is illustrated in Table 5.3. If he has a sweet tooth, there is no reason why he should not have a pudding with his tea provided he can fit it into his daily allowance. When he plays squash, two extra exchanges (a Kitkat, for example) should prevent hypoglycaemia.

DIET AND INSULIN-DEPENDENT DIABETES

Provided the patient is not overweight, there is no need to cut down the amount he eats but it must be evenly spread through the day. It is usual to recommend three main meals with a snack before bed. Snacks mid-morning and mid-afternoon are sometimes necessary to prevent hypoglycaemia.

The carbohydrate exchange system

Views about carbohydrate in the diabetic diet have changed in recent years. It used to be thought that people with diabetes should have a low carbohydrate diet (in other words eat fat and protein in preference). It has now been shown that diabetic control is just as good if they eat a high proportion of carbohydrate. Nevertheless, carbohydrate is converted to glucose in the blood so it is important to distribute carbohydrate-containing foods evenly throughout the day and consistently from one day to the next. To make this possible, the system of *carbohydrate exchanges* is used. An exchange list shows the number of grams of carbohydrate contained in standard helpings of a wide range of foods. An exchange (10 g of carbohydrate) is the 'unit of currency'. So, for example, one-third of a pint of milk, two plain biscuits or a small slice of white bread all contain 10 g of carbohydrate or one exchange. Becoming familiar with the carbohydrate contents of a wide range of foods allows a varied diet.

Fibre and sugar in the diabetic diet

So far this discussion has just considered the *quantity* of carbohydrate. Matters are complicated by the fact that not all carbohydrate foods have the same effect on blood sugar. Starchy foods, fruit, wholemeal bread and pulses are more slowly absorbed and converted to blood glucose than simple sugars. A high fibre diet may improve diabetic control and should be encouraged. Whether foods containing sugar should be allowed is more controversial; it has been traditional to forbid them completely. This has meant that people are denied many of their favourite foods. If the diabetic patient (and, better still, the whole family) can develop a taste for a high fibre diet and do without cakes and puddings, so much the better. If, on the other hand, he cannot live without them, it is best to face up to this and teach him how to estimate the carbohydrate content of sweet things and include them as part of his allowance or increase his insulin dose on special occasions if he eats extra.

Free foods

While a regular carbohydrate intake is the cornerstone of the diabetic diet, protein and fat have little effect on blood glucose and do not need to be regulated so carefully. However, fat is rich in calories and increases the risk of heart attacks, strokes and gangrene by increasing the level of fat in the blood. So it is advisable for the diabetic patient to restrict fatty foods as far as possible and eat vegetable fat for preference (for example, low fat spread rather than butter) to reduce the risk of heart disease. Vegetables other than potatoes mostly contain little carbohydrate, few calories and plenty of fibre so they make excellent 'fillers'. This is particularly important for people with a big appetite who want to lose weight.

Exercise

Regular exercise is particularly important for people with diabetes because it helps prevent obesity and may improve diabetic control (see page 70). However, patients must understand that it lowers blood glucose and may cause hypoglycaemia if its effects are not balanced against their diet and insulin doses. The management of an insulin-dependent diabetic who takes part in competitive sport and advice for more moderate activity has been discussed in Case History 4.2. It is important to explain that even activities like mowing the lawn or digging the garden can lower blood glucose and cause a hypo; but this can be prevented by taking extra food in advance (an extra sandwich, biscuits or fruit juice) and glucose (a chocolate bar or dextrose tablets) if the symptoms of hypoglycaemia come on.

DIABETES AND INTERCURRENT ILLNESS

Striking a balance between diet and insulin is always important but never more so than during an illness like flu or a stomach upset. On the one hand, it might seem sensible to cut down your insulin if you are off your food but, on the other, illness increases levels of the stress hormones and may actually increase the need for insulin whether or not you are eating. Page 64 describes how cutting the insulin dose (and even the most experienced diabetics may find the urge to do this irresistible) can tip you into ketoacidosis. Before David has his next dose of flu, he needs to know the 'sick day rules' summarised in Table 5.4. It is good practice to give every patient a card with this information and advise them to keep it readily accessible.

Table 5.4 Specimen 'sick day rules' for people on insulin

- *Do not reduce your dose(s) of insulin even if you are off your food*

If you do not feel like eating, replace your normal portions (exchanges) with fluids like milk or fruit juice; stir in sugar to make up the portions or drink Lucozade if necessary. Drink plenty of sugar-free liquids as well

- *Measure your blood sugar four times a day*

(before breakfast, lunch, tea and bedtime)

- *At **each** of these times:*

if your blood sugar is between *11 and 17 mmol/l*, have ***4 extra units*** of clear insulin
if it is *more than 17 mmol/l*, have ***6 extra units*** of clear insulin
if it is *below 11 mmol/l*, take **no** extra insulin
Take two aspirin or paracetamol four times a day if you have a temperature

- *If your blood sugars are more than 22 on two consecutive tests*

or

- *You are vomiting and unable to keep anything down*

or

- *You do not know what to do*

Telephone Pat Clarke or Heather Daly or Ward C54 } on Nottingham 421421

- *Don't stop your insulin*
- *Don't guess, test*

LONGER-TERM EDUCATION

Objectives

An important principle of education is that the teacher and learner should be clear what is expected of them. Realistic objectives have to be set. In the early days when teaching is mostly done one-to-one, the objectives are obvious: to master insulin injections, balance insulin doses against diet and exercise, and monitor diabetic control with blood or urine tests. Now other methods of teaching such as books, slides, videos and group teaching can be used to reinforce what has already been taught and to introduce new ideas. Group teaching, discussed in Chapters 4 and 7, is a particularly good way of doing this because it allows people like David and Sally to share their experiences with other young couples in the same position.

Table 5.5 illustrates the learning objectives for a newly diagnosed insulin-dependent diabetic patient in the first 3 months from diagnosis. Some may seem obvious but it is often the most obvious which are overlooked.

Table 5.5 Learning objectives for an insulin-dependent diabetic in the first 3 months from diagnosis

	He should be able to describe
Monitoring	Urine or blood testing, how to record the results and how to adjust insulin doses on the strength of them
Insulin	His insulin doses and the length of action of the insulin(s)
	How to draw up insulin, where to inject it and the care, storage and disposal of syringes and insulin
Diet	Why meals and snacks need to be punctual
	Why there is a need for carbohydrate exchanges
	The quantity and types of carbohydrate in each meal and snack
Hypoglycaemia	Symptoms, likely causes, prevention and treatment
	Sensible precautions for activity, driving, shift work and delayed meals. He should back this up by showing that he always carries sugar and identification that he is diabetic
Illness	What to do in the event of vomiting or other illness
Driving	Confirm that he has notified the driving licence authority and his insurance company
Contact	Who he would contact at times of crisis

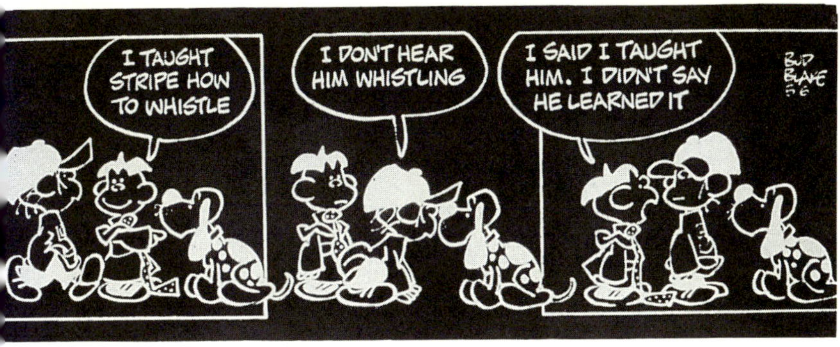
I TAUGHT STRIPE HOW TO WHISTLE
I DON'T HEAR HIM WHISTLING
I SAID I TAUGHT HIM. I DIDN'T SAY HE LEARNED IT
BUD BLAKE 56

Fig. 5.3 Evaluation of diabetes education is essential.

Evaluation

Setting objectives and teaching is not enough, it is essential to check that the patient has learned. Some objectives are easy to evaluate: patients can be asked to demonstrate practical techniques such as drawing up insulin or show that they have glucose tablets or sweets with them. Factual knowledge can be tested by questionnaires and taught again if necessary. However, there is a wide gulf between knowing something in theory and putting it into practice (Fig. 5.3). The ultimate proof that David understands hypoglycaemia comes when he recognises it and responds to it correctly. At this stage it becomes important not to mollycoddle or overprotect him. The best way of learning is to make mistakes. Excessive caution makes a bad teacher!

Lay advisers

The newly diagnosed diabetic patient and his family need a great deal of support. Much of this can come from doctors and nurses if they are willing to make themselves available to listen to their problems and give advice when it is needed. However, unlike their patient, doctors and nurses do not themselves have diabetes. It may be helpful to introduce someone of the same age who has had diabetes for a few years and manages it well. This allows David to see that it is possible for people with diabetes to have good health and an almost unrestricted lifestyle and gives him the chance to pick up tips and ask the sort of questions which he might not wish to bother the doctor or nurse with. Lay advisers must be selected carefully and it is a matter of judgement how soon after diagnosis to introduce one. It is a good idea for diabetes units to keep a list of the names of some of their friendliest and most cheerful diabetic patients who might be willing to help in this way.

INSULIN TREATMENT, OVERTREATMENT AND OBESITY

Case History 5.2

Judith works as a shop assistant and has had diabetes since she was 12. At first she had just 25 units of long-acting insulin in the morning, her urine tests were always negative and she was thin. Between the ages of 15 and 20 her insulin dose was gradually increased to 50 units and she began to put on weight but her urine tests were often positive. After hearing a lecture about diabetic complications a year ago she turned over a new leaf and decided to improve her control; however, she has increased her insulin dose to 90 units and her urine tests are no better. Worse still, she now weighs 70 kg and is self-conscious about her figure because she has found a new boyfriend. She always feels hungry and has to nibble between meals, becomes shaky and sweaty if her meals are delayed, often wakes with a headache and feels generally under the weather. Her general practitioner is unsympathetic and the clinic doctor is more concerned about her HbA_1 than her marriage prospects.

What is overtreatment?

Obesity is a common problem because one of insulin's effects is to build up the fat stores. Some unfortunate people only achieve good control at the expense of putting on weight, but others get the worst of both worlds and are not even well controlled. Judith is getting too much of the wrong sort of insulin, a situation described as *insulin overtreatment*. If she repeatedly attended the casualty department with severe hypos it would be easy to spot what was wrong but the clues are less obvious. An unusually big appetite, shakiness if meals are delayed and a compulsion to nibble at other times are all symptoms of hypoglycaemia during the day; headaches first thing in the morning suggest that she is also going hypo during sleep. Sometimes, fits during the night are the only evidence of overtreatment.

As a rough rule of thumb, an insulin dose greater than 1 unit/kg body weight should suggest overtreatment. Paradoxically, higher insulin doses can make control worse rather than better because 'silent' hypoglycaemia causes the release of the stress hormones (glucagon, cortisol, growth hormone and catecholamines) which protect the body by opposing the action of insulin. This sets up a vicious circle of increasing insulin doses, hypoglycaemia, obesity and poor control.

Obesity and insulin-dependent diabetes

Some diabetics have no identifiable cause for obesity but others have a treatable problem; some common examples are summarised in Table 5.6. Fear of diabetic complications, indirectly, is one. The patient panics if his urine tests are positive and increases his insulin doses. A low renal threshold for glucose (see page 24) is another. Here, urine tests are a misleading guide to insulin treatment because they are positive even when the blood sugar is low. Hypothyroidism is more common in people with diabetes than in others and could cause symptoms not unlike Judith's. Finally, like everyone else, diabetics may be overweight because they are bored or depressed.

Judith's weight problem dates back to her teens; her control was poor then because she had an irregular diet and unsuitable insulin regimen. On once-daily long-acting insulin her blood glucose was

Table 5.6 Treatable causes of obesity in insulin-dependent diabetes

- Insulin dose too high
    - Fear of complications
    - Fear of hyperglycaemia
    - Inappropriate advice by doctors or nurses
    - Low renal threshold for glucose
- Inappropriate insulin regimen
    - Once-daily long-acting insulin
    - Incorrect ratio of long-acting to short-acting insulin
- Eating too much
- Too little exercise
- Other diseases such as hypothyroidism

high during the day and, unknown to her, low during the night. When she increased her insulin dose without paying attention to her diet, she ended up taking far too much insulin and simply put on weight.

Slimming advice for diabetics

The approach is the same whether or not the problem is overtreatment: a suitable insulin regimen, a lower dose, more exercise, less to eat, and a reliable means of monitoring diabetic control. For someone with a low renal threshold, this must be blood glucose monitoring. Doses of long-acting insulin should be kept as small as possible, in Judith's case given twice-daily with short-acting insulin as well. The insulin dose can sometimes be reduced by over 50% in people who are overtreated. This is best done in several steps. For people whose insulin dose does not seem excessive at the start, it might be reduced by 20–30% to allow dieting without hypoglycaemia. It is usually best to reduce the morning and evening short-acting insulin doses. The dietary advice will vary depending on how much the patient was eating before, and should ideally come from a dietitian, but the rules are simple. Main meals are reduced (by 10–30 g of carbohydrate, for example) but small snacks are allowed between them if needed to prevent hypoglycaemia. Lower calorie foods like fruit make better snacks than crisps or biscuits and a high fibre diet is more filling for the same number of calories. Other advice is summarised in Table 5.7.

Dieting is hard work so encouragement and support are an important part of Judith's treatment. Table 5.8 gives some general tips for anyone who is trying to lose weight.

Table 5.7 Dietary advice for an insulin-treated patient who wants to lose weight

- Eat carbohydrates with a high fibre content (such as granary bread, fruit, vegetables)
- Cut down the carbohydrate content of each main meal but take light snacks in between to prevent hypoglycaemia
- Avoid fried foods, butter and margarine
- Cut down on diary produce; use skimmed milk and eat cottage cheese rather than hard cheeses
- Remove fat from meat, eat less red meat and more fish and white meat
- Drink less alcohol

Table 5.8 General tips for slimmers

- Persuade a friend or relative to diet with you and get the rest of the family to eat the same things as yourself
- Persuade your boyfriend or family to sponsor you for each pound you lose
- Write down everything you eat to make you more aware of the quantities
- Drink plenty of water with meals to make you feel fuller
- Buy smaller dinner plates so that the portions look bigger
- Go out for a walk if you feel like raiding the larder
- If you must nibble, chew celery or carrots
- Vary your diet and make the food look attractive; try new recipes
- Plot your weight on a graph and pin it on the wall so you can see your progress
- Do not try to do it too fast; aim to lose 1 kg/month = 12 kg (nearly 2 stone) in a year

DIABETES AND PREGNANCY

Case History 5.3

Lesley is a 21-year-old secretary who developed insulin-dependent diabetes 7 years ago. Her diabetes was well controlled for the first 18 months but then she rebelled and stopped attending clinic. Now she is married and she and her husband want to start a family but they are worried because they have heard that pregnancy is unsafe for a diabetic. She is on twice-daily mixed insulin but has not done a test for years.

Pages 104–8 explain the theoretical background to diabetic pregnancy but here are the practicalities as they apply to Lesley.

Pre-pregnancy counselling

First, Lesley and her husband can be told that pregnancy is perfectly safe. Provided she looks after herself carefully she stands almost as good a chance of having a healthy baby as any other woman of her age. Their baby will stand a slightly increased chance of eventually becoming diabetic (about one in 50) but this need not affect their plans. The importance of good control is stressed, not just during the pregnancy but also at the time the baby is conceived. She must aim for an HbA_1 close to normal and continue the pill until she has achieved it. This should be possible with her present insulins but she will need to take care with her diet and do regular blood tests (before each main meal and before her bedtime snack on 2 days each week). Regular contact with the diabetes nurse will help to motivate her, particularly important if there is a long delay between her stopping the pill and conceiving.

Antenatal care

Once pregnant, Lesley is best cared for in a combined clinic where the diabetic and obstetric teams see her jointly. Blood tests now need to be done both before and after meals, aiming for levels below 6 mmol/l before and 8 mmol/l afterwards. Three times daily insulin (short-acting and intermediate-acting insulin before breakfast, short-acting before tea and intermediate-acting before bed) gives better overnight control than twice-daily insulin and is often used in preference. She may eventually need four injections to achieve good control without hypoglycaemia. Her insulin requirements will increase as pregnancy goes on, probably doubling by 28 weeks. Tight control increases the risk of severe hypoglycaemia so Lesley's husband needs to have a glucagon kit (see Appendix 6). They must be reassured that the baby will not be harmed even if Lesley has a severe hypo, and given day and night telephone numbers to contact the diabetes team for help and guidance.

Apart from supervising her diabetic control, the combined clinic will monitor progress of the pregnancy. Ultrasound scans are used to check her dates and to exclude major fetal abnormalities. Later, measurement of the pregnancy hormones in her blood provide another index of fetal well-being. Towards the end of pregnancy, a decision will have to be made about the timing of delivery; increasingly, diabetic pregnancies are allowed to go to term, but there is still a risk of sudden death of the fetus near to term and labour is usually induced if there is any hint of trouble.

Management of diabetes during labour and delivery

As during surgery (see Case History 7.4, page 165), blood glucose is most conveniently controlled with an insulin/glucose infusion regimen. An intravenous drip is set up and 5% dextrose infused at a constant rate of 100 ml/h through a volumetric pump. Insulin is given from a syringe pump through the same intravenous cannula. Fingerprick blood glucose is measured every 30 min with a bedside reflectance meter and the rate of insulin infusion adjusted by the midwife to keep the blood glucose between 3 and 7 mmol/l (see Table 5.9).

Table 5.9 Insulin and dextrose infusion regimen for the management of labour

5% *Dextrose* 100 ml/h from a volumetric pump
Soluble insulin (diluted to 1 unit/ml); infusion rate adjusted every 30 min according to the blood glucose

Blood glucose (mmol/l)	*Insulin infusion rate* (ml/h)
<4	0
4–6	1
6–8	2
>8	3

After delivery

Even with good control during pregnancy and labour, there is a risk that the newborn baby may become hypoglycaemic in the first 24 h so it is customary to do regular heelprick blood glucose tests; sometimes this means admission to the neonatal unit although it is best if the baby can go to the postnatal ward with its mother. If she delivers in the evening, she can have a small dose of medium-acting insulin and a light evening meal immediately after delivery, reverting to the insulin doses she was on before pregnancy next day.

Diabetic mothers can be encouraged to breastfeed like anyone else but disturbed nights and the strain of looking after a new baby can upset diabetic control so the new mother may need as much support in the early months as she did during pregnancy. She should use a diaphragm, sheaths or the pill for contraception until she and her husband have found out how they cope with the combination of diabetes and a small child and can plan realistically for future pregnancies.

PROBLEMS AND MANAGEMENT OF DIABETES IN PREGNANCY

Perhaps the greatest rewards in the care of diabetes over the last 60 years have come from the management of pregnancy. Before the discovery of insulin in 1922, a young woman who developed diabetes could expect to survive only a few weeks or months. In the unlikely event that she conceived, she would probably not survive pregnancy and her infant would certainly not. With insulin, diabetic mothers no longer died but still no more than one in two gave birth to live infants. In some cases the fetus died suddenly before the end of pregnancy and in others the newborn baby did not survive the first few days of life. Better control of diabetes improved matters but expectant mothers had to spend the last 2 or 3 months of pregnancy in hospital and were delivered early, usually by

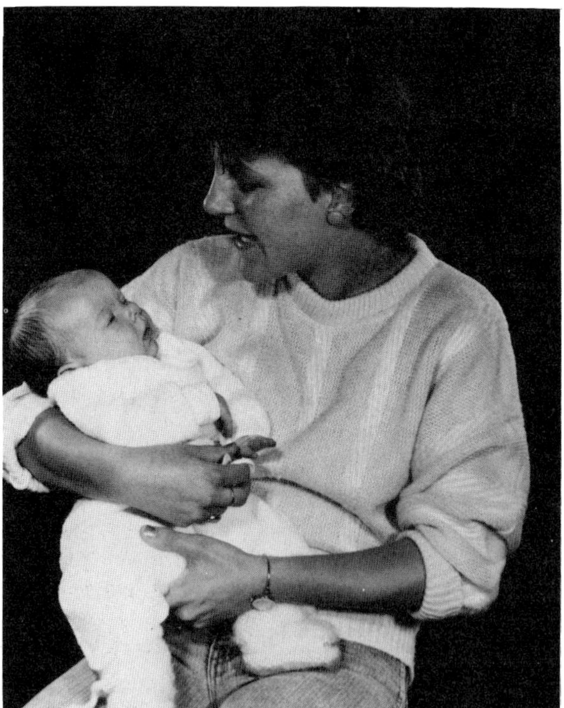

Fig. 5.4 Healthy mother and baby.

caesarean section. With further improvements in medical care, the infants of diabetic mothers are now almost as likely to survive pregnancy and the first weeks of life as other children. However, one major problem remains to be solved: 6% of infants of diabetic mothers have serious deformities (congenital heart disease and spina bifida amongst others), nearly three times the rate in infants of non-diabetic mothers. Poor diabetic control *at the time the baby is conceived* causes this high rate of congenital malformations, so diabetic mothers must aim for good control *before* they start trying for a family. How diabetes is managed during pregnancy can best be explained by considering the effect of the mother's diabetes on the developing baby and vice versa.

Effects of diabetes on the developing baby

Poor diabetic control at any stage of pregnancy is a threat; ketoacidosis, the most serious complication, is as likely as not to kill the baby. Babies of diabetic mothers are often very large, particularly if their mother has had high blood sugars during pregnancy. Unlike her, the baby has a working pancreas and responds to the large amounts of glucose passing across the placenta by producing insulin which builds up its fat stores (see page 7). Though heavy, the infant of a diabetic mother is relatively immature and prone to serious complications in the first days of life. These include hypoglycaemia (the pancreas takes some days to cut back insulin production), jaundice and immaturity of the lungs (respiratory distress syndrome). While these problems can usually be *overcome* by intensive care of the newborn baby, they can also be *prevented* by good control of diabetes from the very start of pregnancy.

Effects of pregnancy on the diabetic mother

Pregnancy is a time of constant change; most relevant to diabetes is production by the placenta of hormones which tend to counteract the effect of insulin. In non-diabetic women, the pancreas simply produces more insulin but the diabetic pancreas cannot do this. As a result, mothers with insulin-dependent diabetes need higher doses of insulin as pregnancy progresses (often increased up to twofold). Mothers with relatively mild diabetes (treated with diet alone or with tablets) usually need insulin, and mothers with an unrecognised tendency to diabetes may develop overt diabetes during pregnancy.

Gestational diabetes

This is the name given to diabetes which arises for the first time in pregnancy and (usually) clears up completely afterwards. It increases the risk of stillbirth and complications in the newborn baby. Gestational diabetes usually develops in the last 3 months of pregnancy and can be detected by a *glucose tolerance test.* This is usually reserved for women with glycosuria, a history of gestational diabetes during a previous pregnancy, a strong family history of diabetes, a previous stillbirth or a history of big babies, although there is a case for doing one in every pregnancy. In practice, pregnant women have their urine checked for glucose and a random or fasting blood glucose if there is sugar in their urine. If in any doubt, a glucose tolerance test should be done without delay.

It is debatable what blood glucose levels should be used to define gestational diabetes; however, if the fasting blood glucose is above 6 mmol/l and the level after meals above 8 mmol/l, many doctors would agree on the need for treatment. The management of gestational diabetes is the same as in women who were diabetic before pregnancy.

A glucose tolerance test should be repeated 6 weeks after delivery and, in most cases of gestational diabetes, will have returned to normal. If it does not, the management is the same as for any other non-pregnant diabetic. Even if it *does*, the mother should be warned that she has a one-in-two chance of developing permanent diabetes and will probably develop gestational diabetes during any future pregnancy.

Management of diabetes in pregnancy

The most important point to emphasise is that good control must be achieved not just when pregnancy is confirmed but *before conception.* Some hospitals run pre-pregnancy clinics for would-be diabetic mothers to reduce the risk of congenital malformations. Whether before or after conception, the priorities are to: (1) monitor blood glucose levels frequently and accurately; and (2) keep them as close to normal as possible.

Monitoring

Urine testing has shortcomings at the best of times and pregnancy makes it even more unreliable by lowering the renal threshold (page 23) so home blood glucose monitoring is essential. There is no room for inaccurate measurements so a reflectance meter has clear advantages over visually read strips. It is best to do at least one test a day every day and a 'profile' (tests before and 1–2 after each main meal and before bed) on 2 days a week.

Diet and insulin treatment

A few women of childbearing age have non-insulin-dependent diabetes. Oral hypoglycaemics are not generally used in pregnancy so, as in gestational diabetes, the choice is between diet alone and insulin. Even if the mother is fat, it is best to avoid too strict a diet because starvation can harm the baby. Eating small meals frequently and high fibre foods may help to keep the blood sugar down after meals. It is impossible to give hard-and-fast criteria, but blood sugars above 6 mmol/l before meals and 8 mmol/l $1\frac{1}{2}$–2 h afterwards on more than one occasion usually indicate the need for insulin. From then on, the management is the same as for mothers with insulin-dependent diabetes. There is more emphasis in pregnancy than at other times on preventing blood sugar from rising after meals. This often means three injections of short-acting insulin a day, with a fourth injection of long-acting insulin before bed (see page 19, Fig. 1.5 and page 132).

Obstetric management

While many diabetic mothers have uncomplicated pregnancies, obstetric complications like hydramnios (excessive accumulation of amniotic fluid) and pre-eclamptic toxaemia are more common than in non-diabetics. The baby's development is carefully monitored by ultrasound scans and measurement of pregnancy hormones. The practice of routinely doing caesarean sections at about 38 weeks of pregnancy is now becoming less common and many women have normal spontaneous labours at term (40 weeks). However, labour may be induced earlier (at approximately 38 weeks) or a caesarean section performed if there is any suggestion that the baby is not developing well.

Problems of diabetic pregnancy

Not all pregnancies are planned and not all are straightforward. Many babies are conceived when the mother's control is poor, in which case control should be improved as soon as possible. Some congenital deformities can be diagnosed by ultrasound scans or blood tests (serum alphafetoprotein) in early pregnancy and the parents can then be offered a termination.

Good diabetic control is not always easy to achieve. Some mothers are unwilling or unable to eat a regular diet and recurrent hypoglycaemia may prevent them from achieving the blood glucose targets discussed above. Some are unable to measure their blood sugar; urine tests are a very poor second best so it may be necessary to arrange for a relative, friend or nurse to take home blood glucose measurements. As a last resort, diabetes can be stabilised by admitting the mother to hospital. However, with a competent and enthusiastic diabetes team and a well-motivated mother, routine admission for the last 8 weeks of pregnancy should now be a thing of the past.

NECROBIOSIS LIPOIDICA DIABETICORUM

Case History 5.4

Jane is an attractive 25-year-old who has had insulin-dependent diabetes since her mid-teens. On the whole her diabetes has given her little trouble, but 2 years ago she first noticed unsightly red patches on her shins which gradually enlarged. Although they are painless, she has become self-conscious about wearing short dresses and swimming and her social life is suffering. She is told at the diabetic clinic that this condition is called necrobiosis.

How common is it?

Necrobiosis lipoidica diabeticorum (usually known as *necrobiosis*), as its name suggests, is the skin condition most typically associated with diabetes. It is uncommon, affecting less than one diabetic person in 100. It may rarely appear in non-diabetics with a family history of diabetes, or in people who have no diabetic relatives and never become diabetic. Necrobiosis may precede the diagnosis of diabetes, develop at the time of diagnosis or, most commonly, appear some years afterwards. It is commonest in young adult women treated with insulin, like Jane. The cause is unknown and it is not a sign of poor control.

What does it look like?

Necrobiosis first appears as small, oval red or brown patches raised above the surrounding skin which slowly extend and may join together. The edges are usually sharply defined but may be irregular and the centre has a red or brown 'glazed' appearance. In some cases (about 5%) the patches break down and ulcerate. The shins are the most usual site but the arms, trunk and face may also be affected.

What is the outlook for someone with necrobiosis?

It usually progresses slowly but may remain very mild or, occasionally, clear up completely. Unlike diabetic foot ulcers (see Chapter 7) necrobiosis does not lead on to gangrene nor is it painful unless it ulcerates.

Management of necrobiosis

To the nurse or doctor, necrobiosis is an interesting and unusual condition; to Jane it is ugly and disfiguring and she is very upset by it. First and foremost she needs sympathy and reassurance that plenty of diabetic patients have necrobiosis and, unlike foot ulcers, never come to any serious harm from it. Injections of steroids into the patches, creams and dressings may sometimes make necrobiosis less conspicuous, but the most practical help is to camouflage the scars with cosmetics which, with skilful application and colour matching, may be very effective. The cosmetics are waterproof and will allow Jane to swim and sunbathe without embarrassment. A demonstration kit is available from one manufacturer (Innoxa Keromask). A handful of women with necrobiosis attend all diabetic clinics and it may help Jane to meet other sufferers. One imaginative way of doing this is to arrange a 'necrobiosis party' to try out the cosmetics in a relaxed, social setting.

Further reading

Bloom A., Ireland J. (1987) *A Colour Atlas of Diabetes*, 2nd edn. London: Wolfe Medical Publications. For a good colour photograph of necrobiosis.

Day J. L. (1986) *The Diabetes Handbook. Insulin Dependent Diabetes.* Wellingborough: Thorsons.

Sonksen P., Fox C., Judd S. (1985) *The Diabetes Reference Book.* London: Harper and Row.

Wise P. H. (1983) *Knowing about Diabetes for Insulin-Dependent Diabetics.* London: Foulsham.

Tattersall R. B. (1986) *Diabetes*, 2nd edn. Edinburgh: Churchill Livingstone.

Handbooks for insulin-treated diabetic patients.

Mann J. I. and the Oxford Dietetic Group (1982) *The Diabetics Diet Book.* London: Martin Dunitz.

Metcalfe J. (1983) *Cooking the New Diabetic Way.* London: Ward Lock.

Diabetic diet books.

The British Diabetic Association print a large range of cookery books. A list is available from: The British Diabetic Association, 10 Queen Anne Street, London W1M 0BD.

6/

Insulin-treated diabetes in middle age

INTRODUCTION

Beyond the age of 30 an increasing proportion of new diabetics have non-insulin-dependent diabetes (see Chapter 7). However, middle age is also the time when people who developed diabetes in childhood, adolescence or young adult life have had it for 20 years or longer and they are the subject of this chapter. Complications like *nephropathy* (leading eventually to kidney failure) become more common the longer you have had diabetes and present some of the most challenging problems. Up-to-date statistics are not available but people aged less than 30 who developed insulin-dependent diabetes between 1923 and 1931 stood only a 50% chance of living beyond age 55. Of course, matters have improved but many patients still die in middle age. That is not to say that complications are confined to middle age or that all long-standing insulin-dependent diabetics are unhealthy. Some who take particularly good care of themselves (or have charmed lives) avoid complications and live to a ripe old age. This chapter illustrates both ends of the spectrum and also the 'grey area' between insulin-dependent and non-insulin-dependent diabetes (see page 13). These are the cases:

- *Mr Briggs gave up clinics years ago because they seemed a waste of time. Now he has suddenly lost the sight of one eye and has a 'full house' of diabetic complications. Is this his fault, the clinic's or nobody's and what does the future hold for him?*
- *For the last 50 years, Professor Taylor has carried a syringe and bottle of insulin in his pocket and had an injection when he thought he needed one. His health*

is perfect but he is impotent; why is this so, and how has he kept himself so well otherwise?

- *Alison James has a flourishing career as a sales manager. Her diabetes was successfully controlled with tablets until recently but now her diabetic symptoms have returned. Insulin is the answer but why is she so reluctant to accept it?*

DIABETIC COMPLICATIONS

Case History 6.1

Geoffrey Briggs is a self-employed builder of 40, diabetic since his mid-teens, who smokes 20 cigarettes a day. He gave the diabetic clinic up as a bad job years ago because he always had to wait over 2 hours to spend barely 5 minutes with an unfamiliar doctor. If he was given any advice, it was never the same two visits running and he usually found he knew more about diabetes than the doctor. He stopped urine testing because it gave no warning of hypos and has just gone by 'how he felt' for the last 10 years. Yesterday, he was stooping at work when a 'cobweb' suddenly appeared in his left eye. By the afternoon he could hardly see out of it and went to the eye casualty department. They told him that he had haemorrhaged into the eye as a result of not looking after his diabetes properly and would need laser treatment; the haemorrhage should clear on its own but there was nothing they could do to speed it.

Now, he is back in the diabetic clinic, absolutely petrified. Examination confirms that he has severe diabetic retinopathy with new vessels in both eyes and a vitreous haemorrhage in the left. His blood pressure is high (150/110) and he has proteinuria (3+ on stick testing) but his blood urea and creatinine are normal. He cannot feel a pinprick over either foot, indicating that he has diabetic neuropathy (see page 151).

Why diabetic clinics fail

It would be easy to dismiss Mr Briggs as an uncooperative patient who has developed complications because he has not looked after himself properly. Remember, however, that he gave the clinic a fair chance and attended for 10 years. He spent many hours in the waiting room when he could have been earning money and what did he get in return? His doctors were inexperienced, he saw none often enough to get to know them and little was achieved in these short consultations. He knew how to 'go into training' to improve his random blood glucose at his clinic visits if not at other times. The doctors increased or reduced his insulin dose for the next 6 months on the basis of this one test, confirming Mr Briggs' suspicion that they did not understand diabetes. Of course, he ignored the dose changes they suggested. Not only was he not systematically examined for eye and kidney disease but he was not even told that he was 'at risk'. No-one suggested that he could improve his chances of good health by looking after his diabetes carefully, stopping smoking and having regular checkups. Organising diabetic clinics is usually the doctor's province rather than the nurse's, but all of the diabetes team can suggest improvements; Table 6.1 lists some common faults and possible solutions.

Control and complications

It is no coincidence that Mr Briggs has developed retinopathy, nephropathy and neuropathy. For the last 10 years he has fooled himself that he is well controlled by 'going on how he feels'. However, his definition of good control is avoiding hypos and he has achieved this by running high blood sugars. Regular urine tests might have shown that he was chronically hyperglycaemic, and home blood tests or clinic HbA_1 measurements would definitely have done. There is little doubt that high blood sugars increase the risk of complications although some unfortunate people develop them despite 'good control'. Once retinopathy or nephropathy have developed, they cannot be treated by improving the blood sugar (though there may be other reasons for doing so) so the aim has to be good control from the start to *prevent* trouble. Before discussing the next steps with Mr Briggs, some background information about diabetic nephropathy and retinopathy is needed (see pages 115–19).

Table 6.1 Common 'pathology' of diabetic clinics

Symptom	*Diagnosis*	*Treatment*
Long waits	It is hard to avoid some delay but your appointment system may be inefficient	Streamline the appointments as much as possible and 'capitalise' on the waiting by having educational displays in the waiting area; a diabetes nurse and dietitian could make themselves informally available to discuss problems
Short appointments	Probably too many people are being seen	Before giving another appointment, ask 'why am I seeing this person again?' and 'do I need to see them so soon?'. 'Pruning' the clinic improves staff morale and the service given to those who do attend
Seeing a different doctor every time	Inevitable unless clinics are well staffed with senior doctors	Screening for complications can be done by a complete stranger; a diabetes nurse and dietitian can provide the continuity and do much of the troubleshooting, and the consultant should try to see all patients every now and again
Learning nothing about diabetes after attending for years and years	(1) The diabetic clinic is an unsuitable place to do all but the most rudimentary diabetes education	Education out of clinic works better; if done in groups, ten people can be taught in the time normally spent on one
	(2) Educational objectives have probably not been defined	As clinic policy, educational objectives can be agreed for the different age groups and types of diabetes
Young healthy patients sitting next to amputees in the waiting room	Sometimes difficult to avoid but an organisational problem	'Stream' patients into foot clinics, pre-pregnancy clinics, evening clinics; if time is limited, designate one clinic session per month as a 'young diabetic clinic'
Bulky, disorganised notes	A common problem of long-standing diabetes	A simple summary problem sheet can save half an hour of ploughing through notes

DIABETIC RETINOPATHY AND CATARACT

Why does retinopathy matter?

Until recently, diabetes was the commonest cause of blindness in adults below the age of 65, and young insulin-dependent diabetics stood a one-in-three chance of eventually going partially or completely blind. Retinopathy can affect diabetics of all ages, even those with mild diabetes treated just with a diet. In general, the longer you have had diabetes the more likely you are to have retinopathy, but older people may have it when the diabetes is first diagnosed. On the bright side, however, laser photocoagulation has been one of the most important advances in diabetes care during the last 20 years, and blindness can usually be prevented *provided retinopathy is detected early*.

What is retinopathy?

As its name indicates, retinopathy (Fig. 6.1) is disease of the retina, the nerve fibre layer inside the eye which builds up images of the outside world and transmits them to the brain. The retina depends on a fine network of small blood vessels (capillaries) to nourish it and supply oxygen. Diabetes damages the retina by clogging the

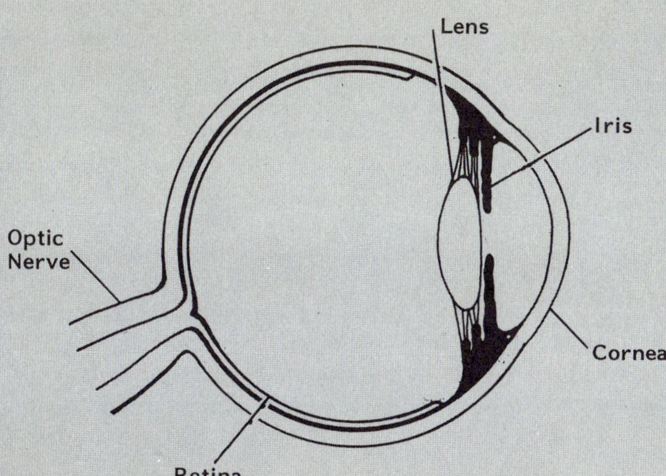

Fig. 6.1 Cross-section of the eye.

capillaries or making them unusually leaky. This impairs vision in two ways:

- Leakiness of capillaries supplying the macula, a small area in the centre of the retina where many nerve cells are concentrated, causes clouding or misting of vision; this is termed *maculopathy* and chiefly affects older patients, often with non-insulin-dependent diabetes.
- Widespread clogging of capillaries deprives the retina of oxygen; this can provoke growth of new vessels within the eye which are fragile and bleed easily.

Bleeding into the vitreous (the clear jelly which fills the eye) is known as vitreous haemorrhage and provokes growth of scar tissue within the eye. With time, the scar contracts, pulls the retina away from its supporting structures (retinal detachment) and causes blindness. This pattern of diabetic retinopathy is known as *proliferative retinopathy* and particularly affects younger insulin-dependent diabetics. This is not to say that diabetic retinopathy *always* causes blindness. Most people who have been diabetic for 10 years or more have some degree of 'background' retinopathy including tiny haemorrhages, microaneurysms (blebs in the capillary walls) and fatty exudates, but only the minority go blind. Some excellent colour photographs of diabetic retinopathy can be found in Bloom and Ireland (1987).

Photocoagulation and screening

While controversy rages as to whether retinopathy can be prevented by better diabetic control, there is no doubt that laser photocoagulation works. A pinhead beam of bright light is focused on the retina to seal up leaking vessels or destroy areas which have lost their oxygen supply. This causes surprisingly little deterioration of vision and can cure proliferative retinopathy by making retinal new vessels simply wither away. Whether for maculopathy or proliferative retinopathy, photocoagulation must be done before the disease is far advanced—in other words before the patient notices anything wrong. Ophthalmologists have their hands quite full enough providing photocoagulation therapy for those who need it, and cannot possibly take responsibility for regularly examining the eyes of all 2000 patients looked after by the average diabetic clinic, so screening is the clinic's responsibility. It is a good general rule that every diabetic patient should have his eyes checked annually. The check-up consists of measuring the visual acuity and examining the retina, usually about 30 min after putting in drops which enlarge the pupil and allow a better view.

Visual acuity

This is measured with a hand-held test type or an illuminated chart read at 6 m (Snellen Chart). Patients are asked to wear their spectacles, if appropriate, and read down to the smallest letters they can manage. If they cannot read all the way down the chart without glasses, this may simply mean that they need them. Asking them to look through a pinhole helps to clarify this; if vision improves to normal, they probably need glasses, if it does not, there may be a more serious problem such as a cataract or maculopathy.

Dilating the pupils

Trying to see inside the eye with an ophthalmoscope without dilating the pupils is like trying to see inside a room by looking through the keyhole. Dilating drops (usually $\frac{1}{2}$ or 1% tropicamide) paralyse the muscle of the iris, enlarge the pupil and allow you to look through the window rather than the keyhole. The patient is asked to look up to the ceiling and one or two drops are placed in each eye. The drops sting for a minute or two and may cause blurring of vision or sensitivity to bright light lasting for several hours. This can make it hard for patients to drive when they leave clinic, so it is best to ask drivers to make another appointment and bring a chauffeur. Some clinics put in a second type of drop to constrict the pupil after the eyes have been examined but we have not found this helpful in our clinic.

Examining the retina

This is usually done by a doctor although there is no reason why it could not be done by a nurse, or for that matter anyone else who is adequately trained and knows what they are looking for. Retinal examination cannot be covered in detail here but is well described by Taylor and Kritzinger (1984).

Cataract

Cataract is the term used when the lens of the eye becomes opaque and impairs vision. Overall, cataracts are the commonest cause of failing sight in the elderly and diabetes predisposes to them at all ages. Cataracts are a less serious problem than retinopathy because removing the lens improves vision no matter how late the problem is diagnosed. Screening, as described above, will detect cataracts because vision is impaired and the cataract can be seen through the ophthalmoscope. Cataract surgery can be done even in the very elderly, and the main problem for the patient is not so much the operation (which is usually done under a local anaesthetic) as adjusting to spectaclcs afterwards.

DIABETIC NEPHROPATHY

What it is and why does it matter?

Like retinopathy, nephropathy is a *microvascular* diabetic complication—in other words it is caused by damage to small blood vessels. In the kidney these are the blood vessels supplying the *glomeruli* (the small filtering structures). At first the kidney (like the retina, see Case History 6.1) becomes unduly leaky and protein (albumin) appears in the urine. Later, the glomeruli pack up one by one, the kidney ceases filtering and waste products accumulate. Ultimately, diabetic nephropathy causes kidney failure and (without dialysis) death. To illustrate its importance, as many as one in four young insulin-dependent diabetics died from kidney failure before dialysis and transplantation were available, more than from any other cause. The appearance of proteinuria is one of the most sinister signs of impending ill-health in a diabetic and predicts not just kidney failure but heart disease, retinopathy and neuropathy. Patients with nephropathy almost always have retinopathy, often proliferative. However, on the positive side, at least a half of all diabetics never develop nephropathy.

Diagnosis and natural history

Proteinuria is always the first sign of nephropathy; it is easily detected with test strips like Albustix. At first, proteinuria is there one week and gone the next (*intermittent proteinuria*). After a year or two it is present whenever the urine is tested (*persistent proteinuria*) indicating that diabetic nephropathy is firmly established. The protein leakage may be so heavy that the blood albumin level falls and fluid accumulates (*nephrotic syndrome*); this may cause swollen ankles, abdominal swelling, pleural effusions or breathlessness due to pulmonary oedema. Anything from 1 to 10 years after proteinuria becomes persistent, the blood urea and creatinine concentrations rise, indicating that the kidneys are failing. Progression to *end stage renal failure* is then inevitable but may take anything from 1 to 15 years.

Nephropathy and hypertension

As well as controlling loss of fluid and eliminating waste products, the kidneys have a central role in regulating blood pressure. This begins to rise when proteinuria first appears and hypertension (sometimes defined as a blood pressure over 160/95) is an almost invariable feature of diabetic nephropathy. Of course, diabetic patients without nephropathy may also be hypertensive, particularly as they grow older.

Treatment of diabetic nephropathy

Hypertension throws an extra strain on the kidneys so it must be carefully controlled with drugs. Oedema may need diuretic treatment and low protein diets are sometimes used in the hope of slowing the progression of nephropathy. Important though these measures are they can, at best, delay end stage renal failure but cannot prevent it. Improving diabetic control probably does not benefit the kidneys once the blood creatinine is raised.

Until recently, end stage renal failure was a death sentence for diabetics because they were not accepted for renal dialysis or transplantation. As resources have improved, increasing numbers of diabetics have been accepted and, in the United States at least, diabetes is now the commonest cause of renal failure requiring dialysis/transplantation. Dialysis may either be *haemodialysis* (kidney machine treatment for several hours two to three times a week) or *continuous ambulatory peritoneal dialysis* (CAPD) (where several litres of dialysis fluid are poured into the peritoneal cavity and changed after 6–8 h). Even blind diabetics can manage dialysis surprisingly well, but whether blind or not the best quality of life is maintained with a successful renal transplant.

Table 6.2 A specimen problem list and treatment plan (emphasising that the information given to the patient is a key aspect of his care)

Symptom	*What the patient is told*	*Other action*
Poor knowledge of diabetes	He is invited to attend a series of informal group re-education sessions with other long-duration insulin-dependent diabetics (see pages 72–6)	
Chronic hyperglycaemia	Better control will not help his eyes, kidneys or high blood pressure at this stage but may make him feel generally better; however there is no rush to alter his treatment	Wait and assess his attitude during the group education sessions, but consider introducing home blood glucose monitoring and multiple injections (pages 131–4)
Proliferative diabetic retinopathy	The vision in his left eye will probably improve over several weeks but he may have further haemorrhages; laser photocoagulation should protect his right eye from haemorrhages and *may* save the vision in his left	Urgent right laser photocoagulation, and consider treatment to the left eye when the vitreous haemorrhage clears
Persistent proteinuria with normal urea and creatinine Hypertension	His kidneys are 'scarred' by diabetes and may eventually fail, probably many years hence; even if this happens, he will probably be accepted for dialysis or a transplant, but good blood pressure control should help to protect his kidneys	Treat hypertension and measure blood pressure, urinary protein, blood urea and creatinine regularly
Peripheral neuropathy; feet at risk of ulceration	His feet are insensitive and he could easily injure them; he is given the foot care rules (see Case History 7.3)	Regular foot examinations with preventive chiropody and shoe fitting, if required
Smokes cigarettes	Cigarettes increase his chances of a heart attack or gangrene; it is not too late to stop	Use the education sessions and 'group dynamics' to reinforce the message and encourage him to break the habit

Realistic treatment goals and preventive education for established complications

Clearly, Mr Briggs cannot be expected to absorb all the facts about retinopathy and nephropathy at one time and the positive points must be emphasised. Remember, however, that his unspoken fears are probably worse than reality. There are so many problems to tackle that it is useful to itemise them and tackle them individually. Table 6.2 exemplifies this problem-solving approach. This is another situation where it may be constructive to introduce the patient to others with similar problems and use group dynamics to encourage him to take more of an interest in his own care.

It is now too late to prevent serious trouble, but the clinic must build up as good a relationship with Mr Briggs as possible because there are difficult years ahead. Hopefully, laser treatment should stop him from going blind. But if it is unsuccessful, there will be added problems for him to contend with (see below).

DIABETES AND BLINDNESS

The whole management of diabetes is geared to helping people maintain independence. Blindness can be one of the worst obstacles to this. Obviously there are psychological and social problems common to all causes of blindness but below are the practical aspects unique to diabetes.

Insulin injections

Whenever possible, the patient should continue to draw up and give his own insulin. Several devices may help, though all have some disadvantages.

Preset syringes

These have two interlocking nuts on the stem of the plunger which are set so that it cannot be drawn back beyond the desired dose. Sometimes the nuts may slip so it is best to glue them in place. If the morning and evening doses are different, two syringes will be needed (and they must be *clearly distinguishable* from each other by, for example, a piece of plaster wrapped round one of them).

'Click-count' syringe

These have a notched plunger so that every 2 units of insulin drawn up is registered by a click. A steady hand and even pressure on the plunger is needed or the clicking mechanism will slip. One can check that the dose is right by feeling the number of notches on the plunger with a fingernail. However, these syringes are difficult to use and the patient needs a lot of supervised practice until he has mastered the technique; many never manage it.

Neither of these syringes can be used to mix insulins so the choice will be between long-acting insulin or one of the premixed formulations of short-acting and medium-acting insulin (see Table 1.6, page 18). Apart from drawing up insulin accurately, there is also the problem with both devices of knowing when the bottle is empty. The patient can work out in advance how many doses he can safely draw up before discarding the bottle or depend on someone else to check it.

Pen injector devices

These are discussed later in this chapter; they have the great advantage of bypassing the stage of drawing up because the insulin is preloaded in cartridges. However (at present) pen injectors can only deliver soluble insulin, and the *multiple injection regimen* (see page 132) demands good understanding and frequent monitoring.

Even if it is impossible for the patient to measure his insulin dose with one of these methods, he may still be able to inject it. A week's supply of loaded syringes might, for example, be left in the fridge by a relative or district nurse. If on twice-daily insulin, the morning and evening doses should be the same if at all possible. Otherwise, the morning and evening syringes must be identifiable by touch.

If none of these methods are practical, the only alternatives are to teach a relative, friend or neighbour to give the injections or depend on a district nurse. Because these options make the person with diabetes dependent on someone else every day of the year and demand great commitment from the helpers, they should only be viewed as a last resort.

Monitoring the diabetes

This depends on the individual. If the patient is severely debilitated and the aim is simply to avoid hyperglycaemic and hypoglycaemic symptoms, an occasional blood glucose or HbA_1 may be all that is needed. At the other extreme, a young blind diabetic patient who goes out to work needs to be able to monitor and adjust his treatment like anyone else with diabetes.

Some blind or partially sighted patients can see well enough to read test strips or the display of a blood glucose meter themselves if they are held in the right position and illumination is good. Others ask their spouse or partner to read the tests; some blood glucose strips are stable enough to be read some hours after the test is done. Audio meters which read either urine or blood tests are manufactured by Hypoguard, who also market a simple device to guide a drop of blood onto the strip. However, the use of such meters requires skill and their benefit is limited to highly motivated individuals who can afford to buy them.

Other disabilities

Sadly, people like Mr Briggs often have other disabilities as well as blindness. Neuropathy is particularly disabling because it impairs the sense of touch and prevents most blind people with diabetes from reading Braille. Renal failure, heart disease, strokes and foot ulcers add an extra burden of general ill-health which may make the difference between dependence and independence.

Guide dogs

These are available to diabetic patients, provided they can manage a training programme that involves walking many miles each day.

Blind registration

Even if it is too late to save someone's vision by photocoagulation, he should still be referred to the eye clinic because an ophthalmologist can prescribe visual aids which make the most of his remaining vision and register him as partially sighted or blind. This opens the way to financial and social benefits, training, equipment and facilities such as the talking book service.

DIABETIC IMPOTENCE

Case History 6.2

Professor Taylor is a well-liked if somewhat eccentric pathologist at a London teaching hospital and has been on insulin since 1929, before long-acting insulin was even thought of. His diabetes is an open secret because he carries a bottle of insulin and a glass syringe in his pocket and injects soluble insulin (sometimes through his trousers) whenever he eats. He is notorious in the medical school because he frequently goes hypo and loses the thread of his lectures; outside the lecture theatre, he depends on his secretary to recognise the signs and feed him sugar lumps. Although his insulin regimen has not changed for 57 years and he goes hypo most days, his HbA_1 is normal and he has no retinopathy, proteinuria or peripheral neuropathy. His first wife died 15 years ago and he has recently married a medical student 45 years his junior. At a visit to his doctor, he bashfully admits that he is impotent.

Long-duration diabetes without retinopathy or nephropathy

Less than one in two people diagnosed diabetic in the early years of insulin treatment survived 40 years from diagnosis; many were severely handicapped by neuropathy or peripheral vascular disease, almost all developed retinopathy and about one-third became partially sighted or blind, so Professor Taylor has done remarkably well. Unconventional as it may have been, his habit of having short-acting insulin whenever he ate kept his average blood glucose levels close to normal, albeit at the expense of frequent hypoglycaemia.

Loss of warning of hypoglycaemia

A fall in blood glucose causes two types of symptoms, those related to the *adrenaline surge* (see page 78) and those which indicate that inadequate glucose is reaching the brain (like forgetfulness, a personality change, headache, double vision, unconsciousness or fits). The sweating and shaking of the adrenaline surge act as a warning and allow the diabetic patient to take sugar before he loses control of himself. Particularly in people whose blood sugars are close to normal, who have very frequent hypos and have been diabetic for a long time, the adrenaline surge may be lost so that the first sign of hypoglycaemia is a personality change which they cannot recognise and respond to themselves. This loss of warning can be such a problem that, like Professor Taylor, they have to depend on someone else to recognise hypoglycaemia and alert them to it.

Impotence

This, the 'unmentionable' diabetic complication, is easily overlooked or ignored because men are embarrassed to say that they cannot achieve or maintain a satisfactory erection or reach an orgasm and ejaculate. *Retrograde* ejaculation (when the sperm passes back into the bladder rather than down the urethra) is another aspect of sexual dysfunction in diabetic men. Table 6.3 lists the causes of erectile impotence. Many drugs commonly used for hypertension cause impotence which usually resolves when the drug is stopped. It may sometimes be necessary to try several before finding one which controls blood pressure without this side-effect. Major pelvic surgery, severe atherosclerosis of the pelvic vessels or endocrine disease like a pituitary tumour can cause erectile failure but these are uncommon and usually obvious.

Apart from drugs, the two most important causes are *psychogenic impotence* and *diabetic autonomic neuropathy*. The latter is discussed more fully on page 153 but, in brief, nerve damage disrupts the controlling and coordinating mechanisms for erection and ejaculation. Characteristically, impotence due to autonomic

Table 6.3 Causes of impotence in diabetic men

- Drugs
  Beta-blockers
  Diuretics
  Methyldopa, clonidine
- Psychogenic impotence
- Diabetic autonomic neuropathy
- Prostate or other pelvic surgery
- Severe vascular disease
- Endocrine disease; for example, pituitary tumour

neuropathy develops slowly and worsens inexorably. Erections are never present on waking and cannot be induced by any sort of fantasy or sexual stimulation, but sex drive is not lost. Psychogenic impotence, in contrast, has a psychological cause and the pelvic nerves remain intact. The onset is more sudden and impotence may be intermittent. Sexual function may be quite normal with a new girlfriend while non-existent with the usual partner, and though unable to have successful intercourse, the man may wake with a normal, firm erection. Libido is variable or poor. Surprisingly, even severe diabetic autonomic neuropathy does not affect sexual function in females although ill-health may detract from sexual energy and interest.

Although his eyes and kidneys have escaped damage, Professor Taylor's impotence may well be due to diabetic autonomic neuropathy and there is, unfortunately, little hope of recovery.

Treatment of diabetic impotence

The first essential is to enquire about sexual function routinely and give all diabetic men the opportunity to say if they are impotent. Those who have not the courage to raise the subject may be immensely relieved to have an opening and feel a great deal better just as a result of talking about it. Nothing is more damaging to your self-esteem than impotence; being unable to satisfy your partner sexually may add a burden of guilt. Men often worry that impotence is a sign of decline and decay in their health.

When discussing impotence, plenty of pauses should be allowed for the patient to express his feelings; he may need prompting or encouragement to do so. He should be asked how his partner has reacted and how it has affected their relationship. If the history suggests psychogenic impotence, he can truthfully be told that there is a good chance of improvement or recovery. This, in itself, may lessen *performance anxiety* and break a vicious cycle of poor self-esteem and poor performance. If the problem is autonomic neuropathy, the outlook for recovery is poor and most emphasis must be placed on how the couple can adapt themselves both practically and psychologically. It is important to see both partners together and, if necessary, enlist the help of a specialist psychosexual counsellor.

If diabetic autonomic neuropathy causes complete and permanent erectile failure and the man is keen for treatment, there are several options. Devices are available which use vacuum to engorge the penis, and constricting bands around its base sustain the erection. Alternatively, men can be taught to inject papaverine (which causes a temporary erection) into the penile tissue. Finally, plastic rods can be implanted surgically to make the penis firm enough for penetration but, because this is invasive, it is best reserved for the severest cases.

INSULIN FOR 'TABLET FAILURES'

Case History 6.3(a)

Alison James, 50 years old and sales manager for a sportswear firm, is responsible for six sales representatives in the north of England and spends a lot of time driving from one area to another supervising their work and introducing new lines. She has had diabetes for 10 years, treated with glibenclamide. Until recently she was very well, but over the last 6 months has lost a lot of weight, become thirsty, all her urine tests are positive and she is increasingly lethargic. Six weeks ago the hospital consultant explained that tablets could no longer control her diabetes and that insulin was the only alternative. To show how easily she could manage, he asked her to stick a needle into her thigh, which she found surprisingly simple and painless. Nevertheless, she insisted that she would stick to the tablets a little longer and eat less carbohydrate (although she was already eating very little) in an attempt to clear the sugar from her urine.

The 'grey area' between insulin-dependent and non-insulin-dependent diabetes (see page 13) is exemplified by Alison James. She is not ketosis-prone and has been perfectly well on tablets for years but now her pancreas is producing insufficient insulin. She needs injections to control symptoms and stop her losing more weight. Table 6.4 summarises the reasons why a person who apparently has non-insulin-dependent diabetes might need insulin.

Table 6.4 Indications for treating a maturity-onset diabetic with insulin

- Ketonuria or ketoacidosis, indicating that the patient really has insulin-dependent diabetes
- Weight loss and/or persistent symptoms of diabetes that are not controlled by full-dose tablet treatment
- Temporarily during
  Surgery
  Illness such as a severe infection or heart attack
  Treatment with drugs such as steroids
  Pregnancy

Why has Alison refused insulin?

Not only is her history typical, but so is her reluctance to accept insulin. An obvious explanation would be that she is frightened of giving injections, but this cannot be correct because she stuck a needle into her thigh without difficulty when she last came to clinic. What is needed is to find out more about her social life and work commitments and to pinpoint her anxieties more precisely. This means spending time chatting to her, something which is impossible in a busy clinic. It could best be done by the diabetes nurse taking her away from the clinic for a cup of coffee or, better still, visiting her at home. She may be worried that the need for insulin means her diabetes has become more 'severe' or, more important still, that she will lose her job which involves a lot of driving. She probably cannot imagine how she will continue her hectic social life and cope with insulin. She may also rather like her new slim image.

Understandable as they are, these concerns are mostly unfounded. People on tablets are no less liable to diabetic complications than those on insulin which should, if anything, help to protect her. She can still hold a driving licence but needs to know the dos and don'ts for drivers on insulin (see pages 129–30). Alison can start insulin as an outpatient in just the same way as David (see Case History 5.1, page 84) and need lose no time from work. Twice-daily medium-acting insulin will quickly make her feel stronger and more alert, but it will be hard to maintain good control with a lifestyle like hers unless she has short-acting insulin as well.

DIABETES AND DRIVING

The main problem is that even mild hypoglycaemia at the wheel can impair a driver's judgement enough to cause an accident. This is reflected in DVLC statistics which show that diabetic patients on insulin have increased numbers of accidents. Accordingly, DVLC carefully control driving licences in people with diabetes to protect other road users. Successful prosecutions for driving under the influence of drugs have been brought against people who have had hypos while driving. It is the responsibility of every diabetic patient to ensure that he/she is a safe driver.

Driving licences: the regulations

Drivers are required by law to notify the DVLC if they become diabetic or if there is a change in their type of treatment. This will not prevent them from holding a driving licence but it will be reviewed every 3 years and medical evidence will be needed to support its renewal. A bad driving record, frequent unpredictable hypos or failure to keep appointments or follow treatment are all reasons why a licence may be temporarily withdrawn. Patients on insulin cannot hold public service vehicle (PSV) or heavy good vehicle (HGV) licences.

Motor insurance

All drivers should notify their insurance company if they have diabetes, or their cover may be invalid. This usually results in a small increase in premium, average 5%. The British Diabetic Association will sometimes step in if a patient is unfairly treated. Insurance brokers can provide competitive quotations for diabetic drivers.

Driving: the dos and don'ts

The role of health professionals is to impress upon patients how diabetes might affect their suitability to drive, and urge them to take every possible step to avoid hypoglycaemia and anticipate the situation which might cause it. The following are rules for people on insulin.

DO

- Notify the DVLC and your insurance company.
- Stop regularly for snacks on long journeys.
- Always carry glucose or sweets ready to hand in the car.
- Stop at once if you feel hypo, sit in the passenger seat, take glucose and wait until you are completely recovered before driving off.
- Tell workmates or anyone else who may travel with you that you have diabetes and explain about hypoglycaemia.
- Use blood glucose monitoring to anticipate and prevent hypoglycaemia.

DON'T

- Delay meals.
- Leave your dextrose tablets at home or locked in the boot.
- Carry on driving if you feel even *slightly* hypo or unwell.

If in doubt, stop, check your blood glucose and have something to eat if you think you are hypo. Do not drive again until you are fully recovered.

DIABETES AND SOCIAL LIFE

There is no reason why insulin should interfere with meals out and an unpredicatable lifestyle provided the following points are understood:

- Short-acting insulin lasts for about 6 h, medium-acting insulin for about 12 h. Short-acting insulin is used to 'cover' extra carbohydrate because it is absorbed more rapidly. The doses of the two can be varied independently so that, for example, 4 extra units of short-acting insulin can be taken to cover an unusually large meal.
- The timing of meals and insulin injections can be varied provided the injections are given 15–30 min before breakfast and the main evening meal respectively.
- Blood glucose monitoring should be used to check whether extra insulin or carbohydrate is needed if the timing of a meal is altered.
- Alcohol makes you more likely to go hypo (see Chapter 4).

Take this as an example:

Case History 6.3(b)

Alison has to take an important customer out for dinner and knows that she will be eating a large meal at about 9 pm. At 6 pm, the time of her normal evening insulin dose, her blood glucose is 8 mmol/l so she is confident that she will not go hypo; if it had been below 5 mmol/l she would have had 10–20 g of carbohydrate, if it had been above 12 mmol/l she would have taken 4 units of short-acting insulin. At the restaurant, she waits until she has ordered her dinner (to be sure that there will not be too long a delay before eating) and then goes to the toilet where she draws up and gives her injection. She takes 4 extra units of short-acting insulin to cover the meal, and is careful to drink no more than two glasses of wine. After an enjoyable evening which has guaranteed her a good order, she checks her blood glucose before going to bed. It is 12 mmol/l, indicating that she slightly underestimated her insulin dose. Better that than driving into a ditch on the way home!

INTENSIFIED INSULIN THERAPY

Once someone like Alison has discovered the benefits of making dose adjustments and taking extra insulin to 'cover' meals out, it is only a small further step to intensified insulin therapy. The principles of this are as follows.

In health, the pancreas monitors blood glucose from minute to minute and regulates it within narrow limits by adjusting the supply of insulin. 'Background' insulin is needed throughout the 24 h with 'pulses' to prevent hyperglycaemia after meals (see Fig. 1.5, page 19). Twice-daily short-acting insulin only provides pulses before breakfast and tea; the medium-acting insulin which is given with it acts during the afternoon and overnight. Intensified insulin therapy attempts to mimic the normal situation more closely by giving pulses of short-acting insulin before each meal with a background supply to cover the night. This can be achieved with multiple injections or with insulin infusion pumps; the possible benefits of this approach are shown in Table 6.5.

Table 6.5 Possible benefits of intensified insulin therapy

- Better diabetic control to prevent future diabetic complications and in pregnancy
- Less hypoglycaemia
- Good control without putting on weight
- Greater flexibility in lifestyle and in the size and timing of meals
- Better understanding and motivation

Multiple injection regimens

The thought of having to give more than two injections per day would horrify most newly diagnosed insulin-dependent diabetics, but as they try to fit their treatment around their lifestyle many see that injections of short-acting insulin before each meal would allow them to vary the timing and size of meals and take extra carbohydrate at short notice. Long-acting insulin (such as ultralente) before bed provides the background supply. This four times a day insulin regimen can be given using the conventional bottle of insulin and syringe, but there are also several devices on the market designed to make it easier.

Pen injection devices

Pen injectors are about the size of a fountain pen, loaded with disposable cartridges of short-acting insulin and have an integral needle (Fig. 6.2). A metered dose of insulin is given by pressing a

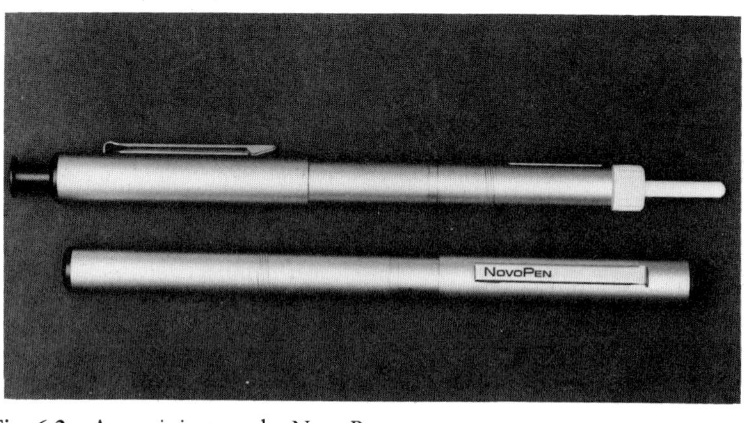

Fig. 6.2 A pen injector, the NovoPen.

plunger or twisting the barrel. The advantage of pen injectors is that injections are quick and simple because insulin does not have to be drawn up each time. This is particularly convenient for people who want to inject without drawing attention to themselves. The gadgetry appeals to many adolescents and may make them more interested in their diabetes and better motivated to achieve good control. Since the pen injector only contains short-acting insulin, the bedtime injection of long-acting insulin has to be given with a conventional syringe.

Continuous subcutaneous insulin infusion (CSII)

A pump about twice the size of a cigarette packet is carried in a holster or on a belt (Fig. 6.3). It contains a reservoir of short-acting insulin which is slowly infused through a polythene tube into a butterfly needle inserted below the skin. The needle is repositioned by the patient about every 48 h and is usually sited in the abdomen. The patient no longer has to give injections, a real advantage for those with needle phobia, although he or she has to learn how to

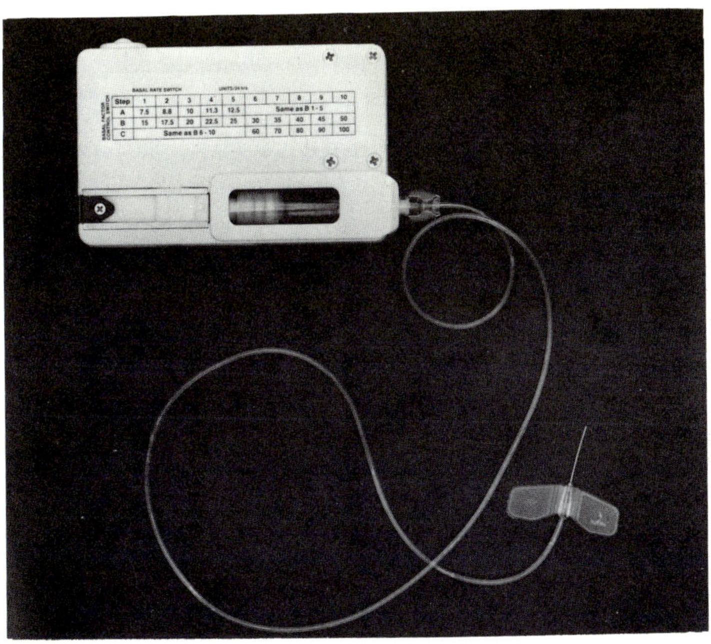

Fig. 6.3 An insulin pump, the Nordisk infuser.

operate the pump, reload it with insulin and resite the needle. The pump delivers a trickle of background insulin throughout the 24 h at a rate that can be adjusted by the patient (*basal rate*). Pulses are given simply by pressing a button on the pump to give the required number of units. Some people find the pump bulky or uncomfortable to wear although it can be disconnected and removed for short periods to bath, swim or make love.

Diabetes monitoring during intensified therapy

Whichever method is used, intensified insulin therapy can only be successful if combined with frequent blood glucose monitoring as a guide to the insulin doses. Urine testing is virtually useless in patients who are aiming for good control because the tests will be monotonously negative if the blood glucose levels are below the renal threshold. Worse still, urine tests cannot predict hypoglycaemia and may be misleading.

Complications of intensified insulin therapy

Intensified insulin therapy, whether by syringe and needle, pen injector or insulin pump, can achieve remarkably good control in many diabetics and give them a freer lifestyle than they could otherwise hope to achieve. However, the following are disadvantages.

Hypoglycaemia

Although multiple injections of short-acting insulin may help to reduce fluctuations in blood glucose, patients who are aiming for good control are sailing close to the wind and may have more frequent mild hypoglycaemia than those with higher glucose levels. Frequent blood glucose monitoring and careful adjustment of insulin doses will help to minimise this.

Weight gain

A major frustration for insulin-treated diabetics is when they put on weight as they improve their control. Intensive insulin therapy is probably less likely to cause this than once or twice-daily insulin treatment, but if it occurs the only solution is to diet and cut down insulin doses accordingly. At least multiple injections make it easier to match up each insulin dose to the size of the meal.

Obsessional preoccupation with diabetic control

Focusing more attention upon control may be counterproductive in some diabetics if they become preoccupied with their tests to the exclusion of all else. There is no simple answer to this except to avoid intensifying therapy in people who are very obsessional.

Ketoacidosis

Because intensified therapy gives more of the daily dose as short-acting insulin and less (or, in the case of continuous subcutaneous insulin infusion (CSII), none) as long-acting insulin, missing out doses or giving too little insulin may quickly precipitate ketoacidosis. This is particularly true of CSII; if the pump breaks down, the needle slips out, the cannula becomes disconnected or the insulin reservoir runs out, the patient may suddenly be completely deprived of insulin. This means that patients using a continuous infusion or multiple injections must monitor their blood glucose at least as regularly as those using once or twice-daily insulin, particularly when they are unwell (see page 95).

Other complications of CSII

Several problems are specific to CSII. The needle stays in place for at least 48 h and may become infected. In addition to pump breakdown or disconnection, there have been instances of pumps developing mechanical faults and infusing at an inappropriately high rate, resulting in severe hypoglycaemia. Finally, pumps cost upwards of £300 and are not usually available under the national health service.

Selection of patients for intensified insulin therapy

This requires good motivation, good understanding of diabetes, frequent monitoring and absolute reliability. Those who are very prone to hypoglycaemia, have lost their warning symptoms, who are unreliable about having injections, live alone, or are obsessional about their diabetes are the least suitable candidates.

Further reading

Bloom A., Ireland J. (1987) *A Colour Atlas of Diabetes*, 2nd edn. London: Wolfe Medical Publications. An atlas illustrating diabetic complications.

Keen H., Jarrett R. J. (eds) (1982) *Diabetic Complications*, 2nd edn. London: Edward Arnold. A comprehensive textbook of diabetic complications.

Taylor K., Kritzinger E. (1984) *Diabetic Eye Disease*. Lancaster: MTP Press. Examination of the eyes and photographs of diabetic retinopathy.

7/

Non-insulin-dependent diabetes in middle age

INTRODUCTION

Non-insulin-dependent diabetes is predominantly a disease of middle and old age. Unlike insulin-dependent diabetes, the symptoms often develop gradually or there may be none at all. Blurred vision is common, occasionally due to retinopathy but more often caused by swelling of the lens which resolves as blood glucose is controlled. Some patients lose so much weight that cancer is suspected. Sugar in the urine suggests diabetes and a raised blood glucose confirms the diagnosis. Background information about non-insulin-dependent diabetes and its treatment has been given in pages 12–13; this chapter translates theory into practice.

- *Mr Jones is newly diagnosed diabetic and needs to learn about the disease and lose weight. Group education is the approach used in his clinic.*
- *Tablet treatment does Jennifer White more harm than good. When should tablets be used for non-insulin-dependent diabetes and when should they be avoided?*
- *Dennis Johnson, a farmer, develops a foot ulcer. Why do people with diabetes have foot problems, how should they be treated in hospital and followed up after discharge?*
- *Mr Green has rest pain in his legs due to ischaemia. Amputation is the only treatment—how will he come to terms with this, how is his diabetes managed during surgery and how should the diabetes team tackle his rehabilitation and aftercare?*

NEWLY PRESENTING NON-INSULIN-DEPENDENT DIABETES

Case History 7.1

Mr Jones is an overweight 58-year-old civil servant. He is persuaded by his wife to see the general practitioner because he is feeling run down and has lost $12\frac{1}{2}$ kg in weight over the last 6 months. The doctor finds glucose in his urine. On questioning, Mr Jones agrees that he has been unusually thirsty and getting up two or three times each night to pass urine. He had attributed these symptoms and his worsening eyesight to his age. Mr Jones is referred to hospital for specialist advice. At the clinic, a fasting blood glucose level of 15 mmol/l confirms the diagnosis of diabetes. His blood pressure is a little high (180/100) but his eyes show no signs of diabetic retinopathy. Sensation in his feet is normal and his ankle jerks are present.

Only a minority of people of Mr Jones's age need tablets soon after diagnosis (see also Case History 7.2). His uncomplicated diabetes can be treated with diet alone. Traditionally, people like him are given a diet sheet and sent on their way with little explanation about their disease. However, they can develop all the same complications as someone with insulin-dependent diabetes (see Chapter 6) and have to realise the potential seriousness of their disease and take responsibility for it. Group education is a good way of achieving this (Fig. 7.1). Mr Jones has no problems that need close medical supervision and is ideally suited for group education. He has to lose quite a lot of weight and will need all the encouragement his family can give. His wife does most of the cooking so she should come to the group sessions as well.

GROUP EDUCATION FOR NON-INSULIN-DEPENDENT DIABETICS

Advantages of groups

A more efficient use of time

Much of a diabetic clinic's clientèle consists of people like Mr Jones. It makes more sense to see several of them together for $1\frac{1}{2}$ h

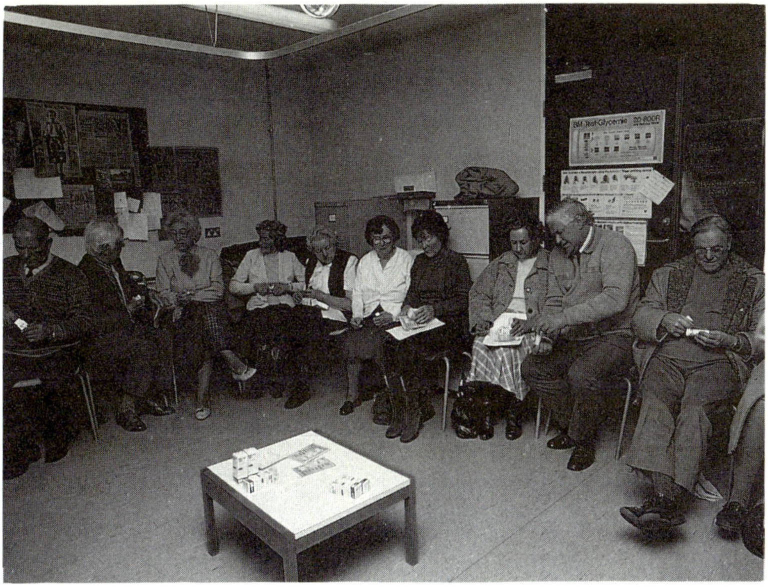

Fig. 7.1 A diabetes group education session.

than to divide up the same amount of time and see each for 10–15 min repeating exactly the same advice.

Emphasis on education

Education is easily neglected, particularly in non-insulin-dependent diabetes because the needs of patients on insulin are often more immediate and take priority in a busy clinic. However, people who have always been overweight and never wanted to be thinner cannot be expected to lose 36 kg unless they understand how it will benefit them. Urine testing will be a meaningless ritual if they are not told what to aim for. It should be no surprise if people report foot ulcers or failing vision late if they have never been warned that diabetes can affect their feet and eyes. If one had to write a prescription for Mr Jones it would not be for tablets or insulin but for a good understanding of diabetes and his diabetic diet; he is more likely to get this in a group than in clinic.

Enjoyment

Few patients enjoy attending clinics. However, some middle-aged and elderly people attend adult education classes for recreation, and diabetes groups can be made enjoyable and interesting in the same way provided the curriculum is presented in a lively and straightforward way.

Questions and answers

Commonly, people are afraid to ask the question that matters most to them because they fear that it is trivial and will 'waste the doctor's time'. A question and answer session can stir up lively and informative discussion which airs many common concerns. Important messages will sink in better than if presented as a lecture.

Group dynamics

The interaction between members of a group can be one of its greatest strengths. Healthy competition stimulates everyone to work harder at losing weight, success is rewarded and people who are struggling are encouraged to persevere. Most diabetic patients have heard horror stories about blindness and gangrene. Being amongst other people with diabetes can help bring unspoken fears into the open, and give the teachers an opportunity to encourage a more optimistic attitude by offering people ways of helping themselves.

Getting to know the diabetes team

The informal atmosphere of a group helps patients to get to know their doctor, nurse and dietitian better, making an approach to them easier if problems arise later on.

Disadvantages of groups

Strong though the arguments are in favour of group education, there are snags as well.

Non-participation

There is often someone who opts out by sitting at the back and not joining in. One simple rule is to arrange the chairs in a circle so there are no back seats. Sometimes it is fear of being laughed at that makes people reticent or aloof. The leader must spot this and encourage them to join in by, for example, asking them a question they should be able to answer.

Domination

There is usually one person who tends to monopolise the discussion to the exclusion of the other group members. Destructive though this may be, that person may have a lot of good ideas. It demands skill from the teacher to use the monopolist as a 'resource' without letting him ruin the whole exercise.

Adverse effects of group dynamics

A group can be supportive to people worried about complications, but group dynamics can work the opposite way if one or more members spread gloom and despondency. People react differently to the subject: one member may be scared witless by it, whereas another may find it helpful and informative. There is no simple answer.

Organisation of groups

Although the educational objectives for overweight patients are the same everywhere, the available time and facilities differ. One possible approach is described here. There are three sessions at weekly intervals, each lasting $1\frac{1}{2}$ h, and run by a diabetes nurse and a dietitian. At the beginning of each session $\frac{1}{4}$ h is set aside to weigh the patients and ask them how they feel; their blood sugar is checked at the final session. The doctor is not formally involved in teaching but is available to see anyone who is unwell. Rather than itemising the content of each session, the overall approach is presented; the learning objectives are summarised in Table 7.1.

Methods of teaching

Breaking the ice

An informal approach is better than making the sessions 'schoollike'. Lecturing should be kept to a minimum in favour of discussion, and there must be plenty of time to answer questions. A video of Harry Secombe talking about his diabetes (one of a series available from the British Diabetic Association) is a good icebreaker for the first session because people are used to seeing him on the television and like someone familiar to relate to.

Table 7.1 Learning objectives for group education in newly diagnosed obese non-insulin dependent diabetes

After attending the groups, patients should know or be able to demonstrate

- That diabetes is a lifelong disease
- Whom they would contact for further advice
- That their type of diabetes needs a calorie-restricted diet
- The difference between theirs and the insulin-dependent type of diabetes
- Five symptoms of hyperglycaemia
- Two foods which contain:
  - starch
  - sugar
  - a large amount of fat
  - a large amount of protein
- Three long-term complications of diabetes
- How urine testing can be used to monitor diabetic control
- How urine is tested and the results recorded
- Daily routine care of the feet
- Whom to contact should they develop problems with their feet and what 'first aid' action they should take
- The importance of annual eye examinations by a doctor or optician and the need to report any deterioration of their eyesight

Imaginative teaching

Making the sessions entertaining and instructive requires resourceful teachers; an imaginative way of teaching urine testing is to get both Mr Jones and his wife to have a go. Since he has glycosuria and she does not, it becomes clear that he should be aiming for negative tests. It also means that Mrs Jones understands the tests and knows how to do them if he is unwell. When teaching foot care, get Mr Jones to take off his shoes to reinforce the messages. Back up the advice with clearly written handouts that he can keep for future reference.

Keeping sessions informal

Stopping for a cup of tea half way through the session is a good way of relaxing the pace and encouraging informal questions and discussion. However the sessions are planned, make them interesting. The teachers must be enthusiastic and approachable and speak plain English, not medical jargon. Do not try to squeeze in too much information in a session.

Aftercare

Time is limited, and three sessions, a bare minimum to cover the most important topics, may be all that can be managed. However, monthly meetings for the next 6 months, run on the basis of Weightwatchers, will keep the pressure on Mr Jones and stop him from abandoning his diet prematurely. Losing weight becomes harder once the first flush of enthusiasm has passed. Suggesting new ideas to introduce variety into Mr Jones's diet will help, and he should be set a realistic target such as losing $\frac{1}{2}$ kg per week.

Diet failure

Not everyone has the willpower to lose weight and even those who succeed may remain hyperglycaemic, in which case tablets will eventually have to be considered. Most commonly used oral hypoglycaemics cause weight gain and, if used prematurely, will undo all that has been achieved; if Mr Jones is put on glibenclamide, he may regain the 6 kg he has lost and lose all incentive to diet. Indications for tablet treatment are considered on page 149.

DIABETES IN ETHNIC MINORITIES

Provided jargon is avoided, there should be no problem communicating with Mr Jones. Not so, unfortunately, with Mrs Swali who is also overweight and newly diagnosed diabetic. Diabetes is up to ten times commoner amongst Asians than Caucasians, and is also common amongst Afro-Caribbean people, so they are more typical referrals to many clinics than Mr Jones. In principle, their management is the same but they pose special problems of culture and diet as well as communication; these are discussed below.

MANAGING DIABETES IN ETHNIC MINORITIES

Diet

Afro-Caribbean and Asian patients may, like Caucasians, be insulin-dependent although most are not. Whatever type of diabetes they have, diet is an important part of their treatment. Their existing diet may be high in fibre but also high in fat, a real problem for the obese. It is no good giving a conventional western diet sheet to someone whose main source of carbohydrate is chapatti. The perfect solution is a dietitian or nurse from the same ethnic group, but few clinics will be lucky enough to have one.

There is no one diet suitable for all Asian patients. Their normal dietary habits will differ according to:

- Where they originate from; people from some areas are vegetarian; some eat only chapatti with their curries, some (like the Bengalis) only rice and some eat both.
- Their religion; for example, Sikhs do not eat pork, Muslims do not eat beef.
- Their wealth.

It is important to know their religion, culture and language (for example, Urdu, Punjabi, Gujerati) and also with whom they live and who does the cooking. It is customary for the eldest female in the extended family to cook for everyone so she must be educated if changes are to occur.

The following common dietary habits lead to obesity: many Asian families eat high calorie snacks (such as *chevda*, *samosa* or *ganthia* which may contain as much as 600 calories per 100 g portion) whenever they have visitors, and it would be regarded as rude and antisocial not to do so. Tea is often made in a saucepan with equal quantities of milk and water, tealeaves and sugar. Large quantities of ghee (clarified butter) and cooking oil are used to give the food its desired flavour; a typical fat consumption in a Leicestershire Asian family was found to be 1.5 kg of ghee and 1–3 litres of cooking oil per person per month. Finally, there may be a high intake of refined carbohydrate in the form of sweetmeats like *burfi*, *jalebi*, sweet puddings and ice cream.

Diet sheets for Asian patients are available through the British Diabetic Association* (an example is shown in Fig. 7.2), and from Brent Health Education Centre.**

* 10 Queen Anne Street, London W1M 0BD.
** Neasden Hospital, Brentfield Road, London NW10 8EY.

Cultural barriers to treatment

To change dietary habits, you have to go deeper than knowing the food value of chapattis. For example, obesity may be seen as a sign of affluence and men may want their wives to be fat. Simply telling someone to lose weight will not work unless you understand the barriers and provide her and her family with a good reason why weight loss will benefit her. Remember that some racial groups have a fatalistic attitude and feel that they have no control over their destiny. They may feel that 50 or 60 is a perfectly respectable age to live to. Religious festivals like Ramadan (for Muslims) impose long periods of fasting and patients may be faced with a dilemma because they have been told never to cut down or stop their tablets or insulin. Anticipating this sort of problem and giving simple advice on dose adjustment helps to prevent hypoglycaemia. Finally, there may be religious objections to beef or pork insulins for insulin-dependent diabetics, although this has been less of a problem since the availability of human insulin.

Communication

It is common for Asian women not to speak English. Seeing Mrs Swali without an interpreter will probably be futile, and it would be best if this were her husband. Even then, one cannot be sure that what is said will be relayed faithfully and vice versa! One could consider using as interpreters other patients of the same race who attend the clinic and speak good English. Whatever way it is tackled, building up a relationship with such patients and maintaining confidentiality are big problems. Books and cassette tapes in different languages, available through the British Diabetic Association and Brent Health Authority, are helpful.

Education

This will almost certainly have to be on a one-to-one basis. Even if you have enough patients like Mrs Swali to form a group, the authors' experience has been that, for cultural reasons, they do not attend.

BRITISH DIABETIC ASSOCIATION

10 QUEEN ANNE STREET, LONDON W1M 0BD

FOOD AND DIABETES

HOW TO GET IT RIGHT

This is simple advice to guide you about the foods you should be eating now that you have diabetes. If you, or a member of your family are worried about your food and want more help, ask your doctor to refer you to a dietitian (who specialises in giving advice on food and diet related to diabetes) at your local hospital or health clinic.

Having diabetes does not mean that your meals cannot include some potato, rice and chapattis. But it is important that you eat less sugar, sugary and fatty foods. In this way you will start to bring your diabetes under control. An important part of staying healthy and having good control of your diabetes is by not becoming overweight and losing weight if your doctor says it is necessary. When planning meals, remember that eating two or three times a day is better than having bits and pieces of food continuously and/or having one large meal late in the evening.

ખોરાક અને ડાયેબીટીસ (મધુપ્રમેહ)

– એને કેવી રીતે કાબૂમાં રાખવું

તમને ડાયેબીટીસ થયો હોય તો તમારે કેવો ખોરાક ખાવો જરૂરી છે. તેનું માર્ગદર્શન સૂચવવામાં આવે છે. તમારા કુટુંબના કોઇ સભ્યને અથવા તમને ખોરાક વિશેની ચિંતા હોય અગર કોઈ જાતની મદદની જરૂર હોય તો તમારા ડોકટરને કહેશો કે તમારી સ્થાનિક હોસ્પિટલ અથવા હેલ્થ કિલનિકમાં નિષ્ણાત ડાએટીશન (ખોરાક વિશે જાણકાર વ્યક્તિ)ની મુલાકાત લેવા પત્ર લખી આપે.

તમને ડાયેબીટીસ થયો હોય તો અમુક પ્રમાણમાં બટેટા, ભાત અથવા રોટલી તમે ખાઇ ન શકો એ માનયતા ખોટી છે. તમે ખાંડ, ગળ્યાં પદાર્થ અને ચરબીવાળો ખોરાક ઓછો ખાવો તે ખાસ જરૂરી છે. આમ કરવાથી તમારા ડાયેબીટીસ ઉપર અંકુશ લાવી શકશો. તંદુરસ્તી જાળવવા અને ડાયેબીટીસને અંકુશમાં રાખવા માટે તમારું વજન ન વધે તે ધ્યાનમાં રાખવું અગત્યનું છે. જો વજન વધી જશે તો ડોકટર તમને વજન ઘટાડવા સૂચવશે. યાદ રાખજો કે દિવસમાં બે અથવા ત્રણ વખત સરખી રીતે ભોજન કરવું પણ ઘણી વખત થોડું થોડું ખાવું અથવા મોડી સાંજે ખુબ ખાવું નુકશાનકારક છે.

Gujerati

DO NOT EAT (×)	EAT (√)	નીચેની વસ્તુ ન ખાશો. (×)	નીચેની વસ્તુ ખાશો. ( )
DO NOT add sugar or gur to any food or drink. Avoid all sweetened drinks, e.g. Lucozade, Cola, Lemonade, Ribena, condensed milk, honey and sweet pickles.	**LOW** calorie or sugar free drinks and tablet sweeteners may be used if liked.	ખોરાક અથવા પીણામાં ખાંડ અથવા ગોળ ન ઉમેરશો. મીઠાં પીણાં ન લેશો જેવાકે: લુકોઝેડ, કોલા, લેમનએઇડ, રાઇબીના, કન્ડેન્સ્ડ મિલ્ક (ઘાટું દૂધ), મધ, અને મીઠાં અથાણા.	ઓછી કેલેરી, ખાંડ વગરનાં પીણાં અને મીઠી ટીકડી ભાવતી હોય તો લઇ શકો છો.
DO NOT eat sweetmeats, e.g. burfi, jalebi, sugary puddings or desserts, tinned fruit in syrup or large helpings of ice cream.	**HAVE** fresh fruit or fruit tinned in natural juice instead.	મિઠાઇ ન ખાશો, જેવી કે: બરફી, જલેબી, સાકરવાળા પુડિંગ, અથવા ડિઝર્ટસ્, ડબ્બામાં આવતાં સિરપવાળાં ફળ અથવા મોટા પ્રમાણમાં આઇસક્રીમ.	તાજાં ફળ અથવા ડબ્બાનાં ફળ તેનાજ રસમાં હોય છે તે લેવાય.
AVOID ALL sweet or cream biscuits, cakes, sweets, chocolate – including the diabetic alternatives.	**BUT** if you are hungry between meals, have a plain biscuit or a fruit.	બધી જ જાતનાં ગળ્યાં અથવા ક્રીમવાળાં બિસ્કિટ, કેક, સ્વીટસ, ચોકલેટ ન ખાશો. ડાયેબીટીસના માટે જે વાનગી મળે છે તે પણ ન લેશો.	ભોજનના સમયની વચ્ચે જો તમને ભૂખ લાગે તો સાદુ બિસ્કિટ અથવા ફળ ખાઓ.
REDUCE the amount of fat you eat by using less ghee, butter, oil, margarine, fried food snacks, e.g. chevda, sevian, cheese and cream.	**USE MUCH** less oil or ghee to cook your meals. Try grilling not frying your food. If eating meat trim off any excess fat. Have semi-skimmed milk in drinks and to make your yoghurt and paneer with.	ચરબીવાળો ખોરાક ઓછો કરશો – ઘી, બટર, તેલ, માર્જરીન, તળેલાં ખોરાક જેમકે ચેવડો, સેવિયન, ચિઝ, અને ક્રીમ.	વાનગીઓ બનાવવામાં તેલ, ઘી નો ઉપયોગ ખૂબ ઓછા પ્રમાણમાં કરો. તમારી વાનગીને તળ્યાં કરતાં શેકો (ગ્રીલ કરો). જો માંસ ખાતા હોય તો વધારેની ચરબી કાઢી નાખો. તમારા પીણામાં તેમજ દહીં અથવા પનીર બનાવવામાં સેમી સ્કિમડ મિલ્ક (તર વગરના દૂધ) નો ઉપયોગ કરો.
USE LESS of the fine atta, white flour and foodstuffs made from it.	**CHOOSE** the coarse (wholemeal) atta to make chapattis etc. Try wholemeal/granary bread and if you like cereals try the high fibre breakfast cereals such as Weetabix, Shredded Wheat, Puffed Wheat, Bran Flakes etc. Remember you need at least one large helping of vegetables and salad every day. Also try to have beans, peas, or pulses, e.g. mung, urad, masur, channa, toor, black-eyed and kidney beans daily.	મેંદો અથવા સફેદ લોટ ઓછો વાપરશો, તેમંજ તેની બનેલી વાનગી ઓછી બનાવશો.	રોટલી વગેરે બનાવવામાં ઘઉંનો સાધારણ જાડો રેસાવાળો લોટ વાપરો. ઘઉંના રેસાવાળા લોટની બ્રેડ તેમજ ઘઉંના રેસાવાળા સિરિયલ જેવાં કે વિટાબિકસ, શ્રેડિડ વીટ, પફ્ડ વીટ, બ્રાન ફ્લેકસ, વગેરે ભાવે તો ખાવા. દરરોજના ભોજનમાં સલાડ અને લીલાં શાકભાજી તેમજ બિન્સ, મટર અને અનાજ જેવાં કે મગ, અડદ, મસૂર, ચણા, તુવેર, ચોરા, કિડની બિન્સ વગેરે નો સમાવેશ હોવો જરૂરી છે.

Fig. 7.2 British Diabetic Association sample diet sheet for ethnic minorities.

ORAL HYPOGLYCAEMICS: WHEN TO USE THEM AND WHEN NOT TO

Case History 7.2

Jennifer White is a plump 52-year-old divorcee who works part-time as an office cleaner and plays for the ladies' darts team in the local pub. After a bout of flu, she feels run down and visits her general practitioner to ask for a tonic. Her usual doctor is away and she is seen by a locum doctor she does not know. Before he has given her much chance to say what is wrong, he tests her urine, finds that it contains sugar and tells her that she has diabetes. Without a word of explanation, he prescribes chlorpropamide tablets and sends her away.

Mrs White knows almost nothing about diabetes except that the lady at the end of the street has it and has gone blind. She is horrified to be told that she has a serious illness but supposes that the tablets will at least make her feel better. Instead, she puts on 6 kg in weight and finds that her face flushes bright red every time she drinks beer. People are teasing her so much that she cannot face going to the pub, which is her main social pleasure.

Inappropriate tablet treatment

Mrs White has the same type of diabetes as Mr Jones (see Case History 7.1). However, the locum doctor made a number of common mistakes and took the lazy way out. He should have:

- Done a blood test to confirm that Jennifer had diabetes.
- Known that most people have heard horror stories about diabetes and provided some reassurance.
- Waited until diet had been given a fair trial before prescribing tablets.
- Asked about her social activities before prescribing chlorpropamide and mentioned that facial flushing after alcohol is a common side-effect (see page 150).

Tablet treatment for diabetes

At least three-quarters of patients who develop diabetes in middle or old age can be safely treated first by diet alone, although tablets or insulin may be needed later. The decision to give tablets or insulin *at diagnosis* can usually be made by answering five simple questions:

- Does the patient have ketones in the urine?
- Is she/he thin, fat or of normal weight?
- How much weight has she/he lost?
- How severe are the symptoms of diabetes? (How many times does she/he have to pass urine at night?)
- Is she/he weak or wasted?

Table 7.2 illustrates how this information can be used. If in doubt, it is generally wise to err on the side of caution and pre-

Table 7.2 Indications for tablet or insulin treatment soon after diagnosis in middle or old age

Insulin definitely needed	Ketoacidosis, moderate ketones in the urine on one occasion or smaller amounts (not attributable to fasting) on several occasions
Insulin may be needed but a sulphonylurea could be tried first	Underweight patients who have severe diabetic symptoms, have become weak and wasted or lost a lot of weight (more than 6 kg)
Sulphonylurea definitely needed	Normal weight or thin patients who have persistent diabetic symptoms after cutting sugar out of their diet
Metformin needed, sulphonylureas best avoided	Overweight patients with symptoms which are not controlled after 2 months of diet
Tablets and insulin should be avoided	Patients with no diabetic symptoms and no ketones in the urine who have not been given a trial of diet

scribe tablets or insulin because they can always be stopped later when the patient feels better. How to start insulin treatment in older diabetic patients is described in Case History 8.1 (page 169).

If tablets are prescribed, a sulphonylurea (tolbutamide, glibenclamide or chlorpropamide) is usually chosen. One common effect of sulphonylureas is weight gain, which is all right if the person is thin but defeats the main object of treatment if she/he is fat. If started before Mrs White has even been told to cut sugar out of her diet, tablet treatment abolishes her symptoms and makes her think that a diet is unnecessary. While this may be true in the short term, it is certainly not the best prescription for good health in the long run.

Metformin acts in a different way from sulphonylureas and has the great advantage that it favours weight loss rather than weight gain; it is best suited to overweight patients whose diabetes is not controlled after a period on a diet.

Chlorpropamide and alcohol flushing

Many people treated with chlorpropamide develop a profuse flush over their face and body within a few minutes of drinking alcohol. The higher the dose of chlorpropamide, the more likely it is to happen. The flush is enough to attract comment and can be a social embarrassment, particularly if it makes the patient look drunk after only a small amount of alcohol. It can be prevented by cutting down the dose of chlorpropamide or changing to one of the other sulphonylureas, none of which cause flushing.

In Mrs White's case tablets were unnecessary. Perhaps she was run down because she was lonely or depressed, rather than because of the diabetes. A few pertinent questions would have helped diagnosis. Even if her lethargy were due to diabetes, advising her to cut sugar out of her diet and express her worries about blindness would have done more good than tablets. Not every clinic or general practice can run groups, but the principles of Mr Jones' management (see Case History 7.1) can also be successfully applied on a one-to-one basis; joining a slimming club may also help. If Mrs White loses weight, stops smoking and has her eyes, feet and blood pressure checked regularly, there is no reason why she should not have many years of good health ahead.

DIABETIC FOOT DISEASE

Case History 7.3

Dennis Johnson, a wiry farmer of 60, has taken tablets for diabetes for the last 4 years. After harvest time the raw area on his left foot which Mrs Johnson has been dressing with Germolene gets bigger. The general practitioner finds that he has a large ulcer on the sole of his foot and sends him urgently to hospital. The clinic doctor who examines him finds that Mr Johnson cannot feel a pinprick over either foot and has lost the reflexes at his knees and ankles; this, the doctor says, is evidence of diabetic neuropathy and has caused the ulcer. In addition, Mr Johnson's blood sugar is high (22 mmol/l). He is admitted to hospital.

Diabetes and foot problems

Foot ulceration is one of the commonest and most important diabetic complications because it can cause terrible disability, much of which is preventable. Mr Johnson's case is typical; he did not know that he should report foot ulcers early (a failure of his education) and was not aware how big the ulcer was because neuropathy had made his foot numb. To understand foot ulcers, some background information is needed about neuropathy and peripheral vascular disease (see pages 151–6). Management of Mr Johnson's ulcer is described on pages 156–8.

DIABETIC NEUROPATHY

Most patients who have been diabetic for 20 years or longer have some evidence of neuropathy (nerve damage). Others like Mr Johnson develop it earlier, particularly after periods of bad diabetic control. Some may even have it when they are first diagnosed diabetic. Like other diabetic complications, neuropathy is partly a direct ill-effect of glucose on the tissues and partly due to blockage of the small blood vessels which supply oxygen to the nerves. This can cause a wide variety of symptoms although many patients are not aware that their sensation is impaired until their attention is drawn to it or they develop a foot ulcer. There are several different types of diabetic neuropathy.

Peripheral neuropathy

The commonest type of neuropathy, it usually starts in both feet at about the same time and then spreads upwards, sometimes to the level of the hips. The hands are usually involved later than the feet and may be completely spared. Peripheral neuropathy progresses over months or years. The earliest sign is inability to feel the vibration of a tuning fork. Later, the point of a pin may not feel as sharp over the feet or hands as over the chest. Awareness of heat and cold and the sense of touch are lost as well. The muscles of the feet, calves, hands and forearms may waste and become weak. A most surprising thing is how much sensation and muscle bulk can be lost before the patient notices there is anything wrong at all.

Painful neuropathy

Some diabetic patients develop severe pain in their legs or arms or over the trunk, characteristically an unrelenting, burning pain which is worst during the night. Painful neuropathy may develop suddenly and gradually improve over a period of months or may come on more insidiously and last for years. It may affect just one limb or several. It usually, but not always, occurs in people with signs of peripheral neuropathy. Simple analgesics taken regularly may control the pain, but it is not uncommon for powerful analgesics to be needed. Strict diabetic control may help to relieve the pain, and drugs such as carbamazepine and imipramine can sometimes be helpful although how they work is unknown.

Diabetic mononeuropathies: sudden palsies of individual nerves

In contrast to the gradual progression of peripheral neuropathy, diabetes can sometimes suddenly 'pick off' single nerves such as the optic nerve (causing sudden loss of vision in one eye), the nerves supplying the muscles of the eye (causing sudden double vision) or nerves supplying muscles of the arms or legs (causing sudden numbness or weakness in one limb, sometimes associated with pain). A nerve affected in this way is likely to recover over a period of months, often completely. Better diabetic control may speed recovery.

Autonomic neuropathy

Another type of diabetic neuropathy affects the autonomic nervous system, the nerves which coordinate muscle contraction in the stomach, bowel, bladder and sex organs, maintain blood pressure and regulate changes in heart rate. Autonomic neuropathy occurs most commonly in people with long-standing diabetes, usually with other complications such as retinopathy and nephropathy. In men sexual impotence is the commonest effect of autonomic neuropathy; at first they may not be able to maintain an erection long enough for sexual satisfaction and later may not be able to have an erection or reach orgasm at all (see Case History 6.2, page 124). Autonomic neuropathy has surprisingly little effect on sexual responsiveness in women.

Autonomic neuropathy affecting the bowel may cause diarrhoea, typically during the night, which can be so severe as to cause faecal incontinence. The diarrhoea may improve over a period of months and then recur. Constipation may also be a symptom. Less common than bowel problems, autonomic neuropathy of the stomach (*diabetic gastroparesis*) can cause intractable vomiting. Bladder problems are also relatively uncommon; the typical symptoms are difficulty passing urine and painless urinary retention, often associated with overflow incontinence. While autonomic neuropathy affecting the heart does not cause symptoms, damage to nerves supplying the blood vessels can cause a large drop in blood pressure so that the patient goes dizzy or faints when he stands up.

Poor control and diabetic neuropathy

Poor diabetic control increases the risk of all types of neuropathy, and better control may improve some neuropathic symptoms, but there is also a form of neuropathy specifically associated with extremely poor control. This might be seen, for example, in a young person presenting for the first time with insulin-dependent diabetes or in an older person, like Mr Johnson, with inadequately treated diabetes. It may take the form of a severe peripheral neuropathy, severe muscle weakness or painful weakness of one or both thighs (*diabetic amyotrophy*). This type of neuropathy often improves weeks or months after blood glucose levels are improved.

CAUSES OF FOOT ULCERS IN DIABETIC PATIENTS

Foot ulcers occupy more hospital 'bed-years' than any other problem associated with diabetes, and may cause endless misery and disability to the patients who develop them. Three problems contribute to the development of ulcers in diabetic feet: poor blood supply (ischaemia), impaired nerve supply (neuropathy), and infection. While all three factors contribute to the development of most ulcers, some are predominantly due to neuropathy (*neuropathic ulcers*) and heal better than *ischaemic ulcers*. Figure 7.3 illustrates the causes of foot ulceration.

Ischaemia

Peripheral vascular disease is discussed in more detail on pages 161–2. In brief, the blood supply to the feet may be impaired by an arterial obstruction anywhere from the aorta down to the small arteries in the feet. The capillary network within the feet may also be impaired, just as in the retina (see page 115) or kidney (page 118). Poor blood supply means poorly nourished tissues and undue vulnerability to pressure and injury.

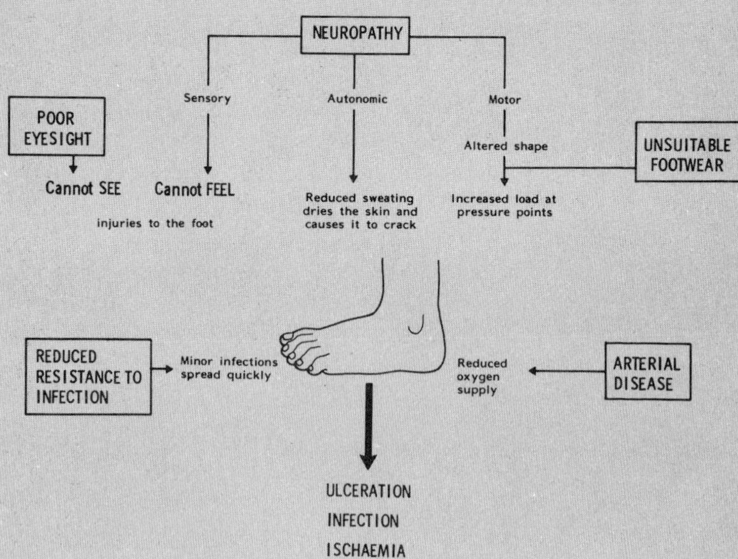

Fig. 7.3 The causes of diabetic foot ulcers.

Neuropathy

Neuropathy contributes to foot ulceration in a number of ways (see Fig. 7.3). Because sensation is reduced, minor injuries or the rubbing of poorly fitting shoes may not be noticed. A hot water bottle or radiator may burn the skin without causing any pain. If an ulcer is painless, and particularly if the patient has poor eyesight because of cataracts or retinopathy, it may be far advanced before he even knows it is there. Neuropathy contributes to foot ulceration in another way: if the nerve supply to the muscles is affected, there is an imbalance between different muscle groups which can cause 'clawing' of the foot and an uneven distribution of pressure (Fig 7.4). This is why neuropathic ulcers are usually found at pressure points such as the base of the big toe. Calluses or pads of hard skin are a warning sign of excessive pressure; if the callus becomes very thick, it may act like a pebble in the shoe and damage the underlying skin and muscle.

Infection

Once the skin is broken, bacteria which are normally present on the surface get into the underlying tissues. This may cause cellulitis (infection of muscle and skin), osteomyelitis (infection of bone), or

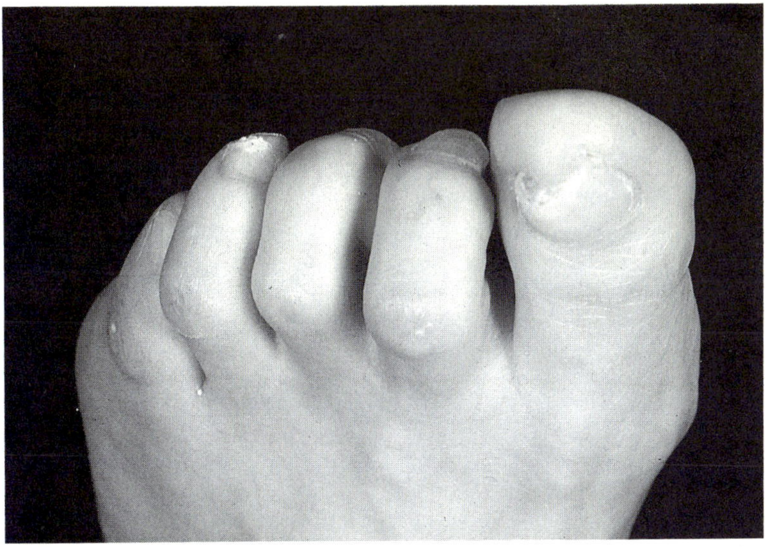

Fig. 7.4 Clawing of the toes due to diabetic neuropathy.

an abscess (a collection of pus within the tissues). The diabetic foot is prone to infection not just because of poor blood supply, but also because the phagocytes (cells which normally 'mop up' invading bacteria) do not work as well in diabetics as in non-diabetics.

Treatment of diabetic foot ulcers

Treatment is considered in two stages: healing the established ulcer (priorities are summarised in Table 7.3), and preventing recurrences.

Take the weight off the ulcer

Some people may be able to rest at home but you may only be able to keep a busy farmer like Mr Johnson off his feet by bringing him into hospital. In hospital or at home, he should rest with his feet up to allow the swelling to settle and take the pressure off the ulcer. His heels should be protected with a sheepskin or fleecy heel pad or he may end up with an ulcer on each heel. A wheelchair will give him a little mobility and stop him becoming bored.

Diagnose and treat infection

The foot must always be x-rayed looking for infection of the bone (*osteomyelitis*) and swabs taken to identify infecting organisms. If infected, antibiotics (such as oral flucloxacillin and rectal metronidazole) are started immediately to cover the most likely bacteria, and continued until the infection has settled and the ulcer is healing.

Table 7.3 Priorities for treating diabetic foot ulcers

- Take the weight off the ulcer
- Diagnose and treat infection
- Drain pus, remove slough and dress regularly
- Improve blood supply if necessary and possible
- Relieve pain, if there is any
- Control blood sugar levels as well as possible
- Insist on rest until healing is far advanced
- Think how to prevent future ulcers and tell the patient

Drain pus and remove slough

Presented with a diabetic foot ulcer, you first have to consider whether it needs surgery. Deep abscesses, osteomyelitis or heavy superficial slough are all indications to operate. More superficial slough can be removed under a local anaesthetic. Many ulcers do not need surgery and there are many antiseptic and desloughing agents available for them. These may not clear the surface completely but soften the slough enough for an experienced nurse, chiropodist or doctor to cut it away at regular intervals until the surface begins to heal. No one agent is right for all situations, and different foot clinics claim success for different preparations, including: Varidase, Sorbisan, eusol and paraffin, and Granuflex.

Dress regularly

More important than choosing the right desloughing agent is to dress the ulcer frequently (once daily as a minimum and up to three times if necessary), best done by a nurse with special expertise. Restricting the number of nurses who do the dressings allows progress to be monitored more reliably. Good nursing care prevents complications so aseptic dressing techniques outlined in ward procedure books should be followed scrupulously.

Remember that diabetic ulcers may take many months to heal. It is easy to become despondent and lose interest but deterioration can occur overnight so regular dressings must continue. See page 159 below for the warning signs of deterioration.

Improve blood supply, if possible

If the blood supply to the feet is impaired, this should be managed as described on page 161. Better blood supply improves healing.

Relieve pain, if there is any

Diabetic foot ulcers are often painless because of neuropathy and it may be possible to cut out the slough without analgesia. This is an opportunity to explain to Mr Johnson why the ulcer arose in the first place and how his feet must be protected against injury in the future. If ischaemia is the predominant problem, pain may be severe and should be controlled as described on page 162.

Control blood glucose

Mr Johnson's high blood sugar was caused by the infection in his foot. Better control will speed healing; he may need insulin for a while to achieve this but should eventually be able to go back onto tablets.

Mobilisation and the timing of discharge

Once the ulcer is healing, the patient can be allowed to walk around the ward on elbow crutches with the foot protected by a slipper or splint over the dressing. Suitable footwear must be ordered at this stage so that it is available when he is discharged. Since many patients with diabetic neuropathy have misshapen feet it is often necessary to supply specially made boots. These should be firm, but not rigid, and spread the pressure evenly over the sole of the foot.

Provided one can be sure that he will continue to rest and his dressings will be changed daily, there is no need for Mr Johnson to stay in hospital until the ulcer is fully healed although it must still be examined and dressed daily after discharge. If it is unhealed and he insists on walking, a lightweight plaster cast with a window over the ulcer may help. The cast must be applied carefully to avoid pressure points which could start another ulcer. If he has good quality, firm footwear, a specially designed insole will help to take the weight off the ulcer.

Management of foot ulcers in the community

Many patients with foot ulcers are managed at home by the primary health care team and never admitted to hospital. Others like Mr Johnson are treated in hospital and then discharged; for them, continuity of care and communication between the hospital and community teams must be ensured. For example, the diabetes liaison nurse might arrange to meet the district nurse in Mr Johnson's home a week after discharge. Diabetic foot ulcers are special in needing to be inspected and dressed daily until completely healed. District nurses might understandably find this a chore but cutting corners leads to amputations. Mr Johnson's district nurse must keep closely in touch with his general practitioner and let him know immediately of any of the following danger signs which should prompt referral back to hospital:

- Increased inflammation and swelling.
- Offensive smell and discharge.
- Increased pain.
- Gangrene or discoloration of the skin.
- Uncertainty or doubt.

It may be necessary to arrange services like meals on wheels and home helps to ensure rest. Flushed with success, it is easy to forget the other foot which is subjected to unusual pressures and must be checked regularly as well.

Good care of foot ulcers in the community saves limbs and leaves hospital beds free for other acute illnesses.

Prevention of diabetic foot ulcers

'Foot consciousness' should start at first contact with the diabetic clinic and the messages must be repeated over and over again. Written instructions in the form of a foot care guide are important as well as verbal instruction and other methods of teaching such as posters prominently displayed in the clinic and video education. Table 7.4 summarises the foot care rules. These must be re-emphasised when Mr Johnson is discharged; meticulous foot care, regular chiropody and frequent examination by a doctor or nurse will be essential to prevent future ulcers.

Table 7.4 Rules for preventing diabetic foot ulcers

- Inspect the skin of your feet and between the toes regularly using a mirror if necessary
- Wash your feet daily and dry carefully between your toes
- Trim nails regularly and have calluses treated by a qualified chiropodist
- Never walk barefoot
- Always check the temperature of a hot water bottle against your face or chest; *never* toast your feet in front of a fire
- Never wear poorly fitting shoes; break in new shoes gradually
- Consult your doctor or nurse at the first sign of trouble

DIABETIC PERIPHERAL VASCULAR DISEASE

Case History 7.4(a)

Mr Green is a retired miner who lives with his wife in a three-bedroomed council house. He has smoked 30 cigarettes a day for 40 years and has tablet-treated diabetes. He comes to casualty complaining of a painful right foot. The trouble started 4 months ago with a cramp-like pain in the right calf after walking the dog for about a kilometre. Since then he has had to stop and let the pain subside after shorter and shorter distances, and now his foot is painful even at rest and keeping him awake at night. The toes of his right foot are a dusky red colour and the casualty officer can feel no pulses in either leg. He explains to Mr Green that his toes are painful because not enough blood is reaching them. He arranges admission to a surgical ward.

Mr Green's history is all too typical. He has continued to smoke despite being diabetic and has severe peripheral vascular disease. If it is not possible to do vascular surgery to save his leg, he will need an amputation. Peripheral vascular disease and how it is diagnosed are illustrated in Fig. 7.5 and described on pages 161–2.

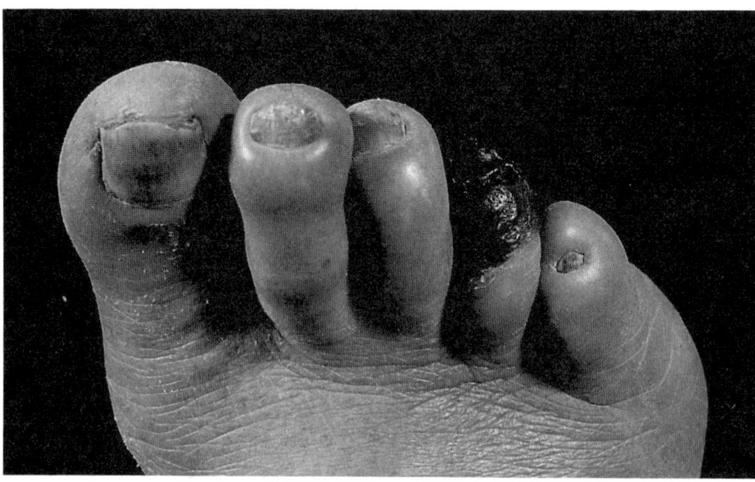

Fig. 7.5 An ischaemic diabetic foot with a gangrenous toe.

PERIPHERAL VASCULAR DISEASE AND DIABETES

Arteriosclerosis, or hardening of the arteries, is one of the commonest diseases and the main cause of death in western civilisation. It becomes more common with age and tends to run in families, but diabetes and smoking greatly accelerate the process. Arteriosclerosis mainly affects the arteries supplying the brain (stroke), coronary arteries (myocardial infarction, see Case History 8.1) and legs, discussed here.

Diabetes causes diffuse changes in the arterial tree from the aorta down to the feet. At first the pulses in the feet and behind the knee become faint and then impalpable, but there may be no symptoms. When the arteries are so clogged that the muscles are not receiving enough oxygen, pain begins. At first, it is only noticeable after exercise and is relieved by resting for a few minutes (*intermittent claudication*) but later the pain is present even at rest (*rest pain*). Claudication pain is first felt in the calves but later involves the buttocks, thigh and foot. Rest pain is often worst in the foot.

Investigation and treatment

Even at the stage of intermittent claudication, stopping smoking can improve the symptoms; in non-smokers, they may improve spontaneously. Persistent severe claudication or rest pain can only be treated by improving the blood supply. First it is necessary to assess the state of the arteries. This is done by injecting a radio-opaque dye into the aorta and taking x-rays (*arteriography*). If there is localised obstruction above the level of the knee, it may be possible to 'stretch' it with a small balloon catheter passed down the artery (*balloon angioplasty*). More often, a length of vein is used to bypass the obstruction (*femoropopliteal bypass graft*) or the lining of the iliac vessels may literally be scooped out (*endarterectomy*). Sadly, however, diabetic patients often have such widespread disease that bypassing one obstruction does not help because there are others lower down (*poor runoff*).

If surgery is impossible or does not relieve pain, amputation is the only alternative. This may be done at any level from the forefoot to the thigh, depending on the level of the obstruction. Of course, the main consideration is to amputate high enough to ensure healing; however, the lower the amputation, the easier it will be for the patient to walk with an artificial limb.

Analgesia for ischaemic pain

Surgery may be the long-term solution but Mr Green's immediate need is pain relief; he has not slept properly for 2 weeks. Few pains are more severe and unrelenting than ischaemia, and powerful analgesics are often needed although milder drugs should be tried first. Frequent dosing is most important; it is useless to give a large dose every 6 h which makes the patient feel sleepy and nauseated for a short time but then wears off before the next dose is due. If a dose of paracetamol or aspirin every 3 h is insufficient, more potent oral preparations such as buprenorphine or dihydrocodeine can be substituted; only if this fails should oral morphine or injected pethidine or diamorphine be used. Pain at night can be particularly troublesome, in which case slow release oral morphine or oxycodone suppositories sometimes work for long enough to allow undisturbed sleep.

Amputation

Case History 7.4(b)

Mr Green's pain is controlled with regular oral dihydrocodeine but his arteriogram shows such severe arterial disease below the knee that bypass surgery is impossible. A below-knee amputation is the only long-term solution to his pain. He is still smoking heavily. It is obviously too late to save his right leg but he is reminded that his left leg will be in danger if he continues to smoke.

Psychological preparation

To be told that your leg has to be amputated is devastating. However, someone who has endured ischaemic pain for several weeks may be so desperate for pain relief that he takes the news surprisingly well. He must be given the opportunity to discuss his feelings with members of the team and his family should be involved early. Patients may reasonably fear that they will no longer be wanted or accepted because they are not physically whole. They may also fear that simple pleasures like going to the pub and doing odd jobs about the house will no longer be possible.

Arranging a visit from someone who has had an amputation and copes well with an artificial limb may be reassuring. For example, a visit from an amputee who shares Mr Green's passion for gardening and has been able to continue his hobby would give him a little encouragement. Most people think that artificial limbs are heavy and difficult to use so just to see one may be valuable. The staff of the limb-fitting service are often keen to be involved early and may like to visit even before the operation. The time needed to come to terms with an amputation varies so it is important that staff treat each patient as an individual with individual fears about the future.

Preoperative care

Mr Green smoked heavily until he was admitted to hospital so regular chest physiotherapy will be needed to prevent a postoperative chest infection. The management of diabetes during surgery is discussed in more detail on pages 165–7. Briefly, he should have his last dose of oral hypoglycaemics on the evening before his operation, fast from midnight and have a glucose and insulin infusion on the morning of surgery so that he arrives in theatre with a normal blood glucose.

One point to be emphasised above all others is that his *left* foot is very vulnerable. Careless positioning while he is unconscious or drowsy could cause a pressure ulcer that might lead to a second amputation. A fleecy heel pad worn during the operation will help to protect his left foot.

Postoperative care

The priorities are summarised in Table 7.5; typically, Mr Green might be treated with twice-daily subcutaneous insulin for several days postoperatively but he must be told that this is just a temporary measure or he may worry unnecessarily. *Phantom pain* (pain in the missing leg) commonly starts a day or two after the operation. This is treated with liberal analgesia and an assurance that it often improves within days. If all goes well, the stitches can be removed 10 days after the operation.

Do not wait until the last minute to make arrangements for discharge. Ideally, an occupational therapist and physiotherapist should visit Mr Green's home. To start with, he may have to sleep downstairs but this should only be until he is confident enough

Table 7.5 Priorities for care after amputation in a diabetic patient

- Maintaining good diabetic control
- Regular dressings with close observation for signs of infection
- Good positioning to prevent pressure on the stump and contractures
- Encouraging mobility as soon as possible (ideally day 2 or 3) with the help of a walking frame
- Meticulous observation and care of the other foot to prevent pressure sores
- Assessing the patient's home to see what alterations are needed well before discharge
- Arranging fitting of an artificial limb
- Ordering a wheelchair

with an artificial leg to manage the stairs. Even while he is convalescing from the operation and wheelchair-bound, a weekend at home will boost his morale.

Rehabilitation

An artificial limb cannot be fitted until Mr Green has got over the operation and the stump has healed but the staff of artificial limb and appliance centres often like to assess progress soon after the operation. The first appointment at the centre is usually 3–6 weeks later. There is no need to keep Mr Green in hospital until the limb is fitted provided his home is suitable, there is plenty of home support and he is fit enough to be discharged.

Other priorities for long-term care

Care of the remaining foot is of paramount importance after an amputation. Often it is misshapen because of neuropathy and a special shoe is needed. The patient or his wife should examine the foot carefully each day and he should visit a chiropodist regularly. The limb and appliance centre will follow progress with the artificial limb but the ward can help Mr and Mrs Green as well by encouraging them to ring and discuss any problems. Even if Mr Green succeeded in giving up smoking while he was in hospital, he may be tempted to restart when he is bored and frustrated at home. Advice which may help is summarised on page 172. Perhaps the most important step is to enlist the family's help and, if they smoke, get them to stop too.

THE MANAGEMENT OF DIABETES DURING SURGERY

A medical or surgical ward in a busy hospital will see someone with diabetes having a general anaesthetic at least once a fortnight. Managing the diabetes is easy if you take care, and yet it is remarkably often messed up. The principles are straightforward. Anaesthesia and surgery have two effects: not eating will tend to lower blood glucose but the stress of even minor surgery will tend to raise it. One cannot predict the net effect in an individual so the ideal approach is to trickle in 5% dextrose, do frequent bedside blood tests and infuse insulin at a variable rate to keep blood glucose between 4 and 8 mmol/l.

The day before

It is best to admit at least 24 h before surgery and do blood tests before breakfast, lunch, tea and the bedtime snack. Monitoring the urine for glucose is not essential (unless the equipment to do bedside blood tests is unavailable) but checking the urine for ketones postoperatively is important.

On the day

If at all possible, diabetics should be first on the operating list (so that the timing of surgery is predictable) and on a morning list (so that their immediate postoperative care is during normal working hours).

Advice given to doctors in our hospital

Morning surgery

Fast from midnight and measure blood glucose at 8 am. If:

- the patient is not usually on insulin;
- anaesthesia is unlikely to last more than 45 min;
- the 8 am blood glucose is between 4 and 10 mmol/l;

you need take no action; otherwise start an insulin/glucose infusion (see below).

Afternoon surgery

Measure blood glucose at 6 and 10 am.

Allow a light breakfast; if the patient is *normally on oral hypo-*

glycaemics, withhold them and give 8 units soluble insulin 15 min before it. If *normally on insulin*, give 8 units or half the usual morning dose of soluble, whichever is the greater.

If any blood test is above 10 mmol/l start the insulin/glucose infusion. Otherwise, decide at 12 midday whether or not to start the infusion as described for morning surgery (see above).

Insulin/glucose regimen

Dextrose 5% — Infuse 500 ml every 4 h but stop if blood glucose >10 mmol/l.

Insulin — Make 50 units of soluble insulin up to a volume of 50 ml with normal saline in a 50 ml syringe; run it from a syringe pump through the same cannula as the dextrose

Sliding scale

Blood glucose (mmol/l)	*Insulin infusion* (units/h)
<4	0
4–7	1
7.1–10	2
10.1–13	2 *and* stop glucose
13.1–20	4
20+	8 *and* call physician

Blood tests — Do them at least hourly to start with, then every 2 or 4 h if blood sugar is stable between 4 and 10 mmol/l.

Postoperative regimen

Check blood glucose immediately on return to the ward and monitor it at least every 4 h, even if insulin is not needed. Check all urine for ketones.

Continue insulin/glucose infusion until the patient can eat, then resume normal insulin; patients who are normally on oral hypoglycaemics and are able to eat an evening meal on the day of surgery should have 10 units of soluble insulin before it with half their normal dose of oral hypoglycaemics and resume normal treatment the next day.

If the blood sugar is consistently above 10 mmol/l and/or there is moderate to heavy ketonuria, call a physician

Further reading

Day J. L. (1986) *The Diabetes Handbook. Non Insulin-dependent Diabetes*. Wellingborough: Thorsons. A guide to non-insulin-dependent diabetes for patients.

Keen H., Jarrett R. J. (eds) (1982) *Diabetic Complications*, 2nd edn. London: Edward Arnold. Diabetic neuropathy and peripheral vascular disease.

Singh S. (1987) *Coping with the Amputation of a Leg*. Available from the British Diabetic Association, 10 Queen Anne Street, London W1M 0BQ. Amputation.

Mann J. I. and the Oxford Dietetic Group (1982) *The Diabetics Diet Book*. London: Martin Dunitz. Diets for non-insulin-dependent diabetes.

Wise P. H. (1983) *Knowing about Diabetes for Non-insulin Dependent Diabetes*. London: Foulsham. A guide to non-insulin-dependent diabetes for patients.

8/

Diabetes in the elderly

HOW COMMON IS IT?

More than half of all diabetic patients are aged over 65. Most are treated with a diet or tablets and many never come near hospital. People often describe non-insulin-dependent diabetes as 'mild', but this is misleading because its effects can sometimes be far from mild. Even someone whose diabetes is well controlled with a diet is at risk of a heart attack, stroke, foot ulcer or gangrene. Retinopathy affects the elderly as it does young diabetics, and it may be a diabetic complication which first takes the older patient to a doctor. How can complications develop before someone is even known to be diabetic? The answer is that they have been diabetic much longer than is realised. Hyperglycaemic symptoms may not have been recognised; vague ill-health, weight loss and thirst are easy to put down to 'old age', and some old people may be asymptomatic even when markedly hyperglycaemic.

Ketoacidosis (see page 64) is usually thought of as a problem of younger diabetics, yet as many as a quarter of admissions to hospital for hyperglycaemic coma are in patients over age 65. Nearly half of these older patients die compared with less than one patient in ten below age 65. This high death rate is partly because hyperglycaemic coma in the elderly may be triggered off by a serious illness such as a heart attack or stroke, but also because the elderly cannot withstand serious illness as well as younger people and may not complain until they are desperately ill.

It is usual to aim for as good control as possible to prevent long-term complications in younger diabetic patients, but this becomes less important the older you are and the shorter your life expectancy. It may be quite enough of a challenge to keep an elderly person free from symptoms of both hypoglycaemia and hyperglycaemia and able to enjoy independent life for their last few years. Treatment, monitoring and diet have to be as simple as possible.

This is particularly true of people who are forgetful or confused, dependent on others, or living in institutions where the staff may be ignorant and frightened of diabetes. This chapter illustrates some of the problems that may arise in the elderly.

- *Joseph Brown suddenly becomes unwell; how can you tell whether this is due to his diabetes and how do you tell the difference between hypoglycaemia and hyperglycaemia? It turns out that he has had a 'silent' heart attack and is hyperglycaemic.*
- *Miss Hardy seems to be going 'senile'. Her real problem is poorly controlled diabetes and she needs insulin. How should insulin treatment be started and monitored in the elderly and what about a diet?*
- *Mrs Sutton has a stroke and can no longer live at home so she goes to an old people's home. What practical help do the staff of the home need and what should they be told?*

MYOCARDIAL INFARCTION AND LOSS OF DIABETIC CONTROL

Case History 8.1(a)

Joseph Brown is a retired butcher, diabetic and on glibenclamide for 5 years, who never used to bother with urine tests and seldom kept clinic appointments. At the age of 69 he is 12 kg overweight and smokes 40 cigarettes a day despite having been advised to stop. For 3 days he has been feeling tired, weak, thirsty and generally unwell. His wife is so worried that she contacts their general practitioner who comes to see him at home.

Distinguishing hyperglycaemia from hypoglycaemia

When someone with diabetes is unwell, the first step is to decide if their diabetes is responsible and, if so, whether they are hypoglycaemic or hyperglycaemic. This may be obvious from the symptoms; some useful clues are shown in Table 8.1. If there is doubt a blood test clinches it; this can be done with a test strip and a drop

Table 8.1 How to distinguish hypoglycaemia from hyperglycaemia as a cause of drowsiness or coma

	Hypoglycaemia	*Hyperglycaemia*
Type of treatment	Insulin or sulphonylurea*	May be diet alone, tablets or insulin
Onset	Usually sudden; often over minutes	More gradual, over hours or days
Helpful symptoms and signs	Profuse sweating Pallor Confusion or aggression	Thirst and polyuria Vomiting
Unhelpful symptoms	Drowsiness, lethargy and weakness may occur with either	
Urine test	Unhelpful	Invariably strongly positive for glucose; ketones may be present
Blood glucose	Less than 3 mmol/l	Above 13 mmol/l

* Usually chlorpropamide or glibenclamide; see page 22 for a fuller list.

of blood, even in Mr Brown's home (Appendix 5). A urine test is much less useful because it can neither detect hypoglycaemia nor give any idea how high the blood glucose is. A urine test for ketones is helpful if it is strongly positive (indicating ketoacidosis) but a negative test does not help one way or another; it is possible for older patients to have severe hyperglycaemic coma without ketones in the urine (see hyperosmolar non-ketotic coma, page 64).

Mr Brown's symptoms suggest hyperglycaemia and this can easily be confirmed by a fingerprick blood glucose test. A diabetic patient as ill as he is needs immediate admission to hospital. On arrival, the first priorities are to assess how badly out of control is his diabetes and start treatment. Blood should be sent to the laboratory for glucose, urea and electrolyte estimations; with a history like his, the blood glucose may be extremely high (60 mmol/l), and the blood urea will also be high indicating dehydration. He needs intravenous insulin and saline urgently (see page 66).

What causes diabetes to go out of control suddenly?

It is not enough to diagnose severe hyperglycaemia, it is essential to look for an underlying cause (Table 8.2).

Table 8.2 Common causes of severe hyperglycaemia in older patients

- Chest or urinary tract infection, viral illness, septicaemia or meningitis
- Heart attack
- Stroke
- Infected or gangrenous foot
- Acute abdomen: pancreatitis, perforated stomach or gangrenous bowel
- Inadequate treatment: for example, unrecognised need for insulin
- Mistakes with insulin or tablets: for example, wrong doses or omitting insulin when unwell

In about half of all cases, no cause can be found

Case History 8.1(b)

After a thorough physical examination, Mr Brown has an ECG, chest x-ray, blood and urine cultures. The diagnosis is easy: the ECG shows signs of a recent heart attack. This occurred 'silently' several days ago and threw his diabetes out of control.

Older people in general, and those with diabetes in particular, may have heart attacks without any typical symptoms like chest pain, breathlessness or palpitations. Heart attacks are common in adult diabetics of all ages and should always be considered if their diabetes suddenly goes out of control. Over 30% of diabetic patients admitted to hospital with a heart attack die, about twice the mortality in non-diabetics of the same age. The mortality is so high because diabetics usually have more severe coronary artery disease than non-diabetics of the same age making them more likely to go into heart failure and develop serious arrhythmias such as ventricular fibrillation.

Care of the diabetic patient with a heart attack

Mr Brown needs close observation on an intensive care or coronary care unit. Although he is dehydrated, intravenous saline will have to be given cautiously because it is easy to precipitate heart failure after a heart attack. The drip and insulin infusion can be taken down once his blood sugar has been brought back to normal and he is no longer dehydrated. Rather than restarting tablets, he should be treated temporarily with twice-daily insulin because diabetes may be harder to control during acute illness than at other times. Do not forget how frightened many diabetic patients are of 'the needle'; perhaps the reason Mr Brown missed so many clinic appointments in the past was his fear that he would be started on insulin injections. A perceptive nurse foreseeing that injections would add to his worries on the coronary care unit could put his mind at rest by explaining that they were just a temporary measure until he had got over his heart attack. If he is fortunate enough to make a good recovery, he can be moved to a general medical ward after 2–3 days. At first he can be allowed to sit out of bed and then gradually to walk around the ward.

Advice and follow-up after a heart attack

Diet

When Mr Brown is ready to go home, what advice does he need? He has not followed a diet for several years, but will be in a much more receptive frame of mind after his heart attack, so this is a good time for the dietitian to spend some time with him and his wife. To prevent further heart attacks, it is important for him to lose weight, eat less animal fat and keep his diabetes well controlled; but by far the most important step is to stop smoking.

Stopping smoking

Stopping smoking reduces the chances not just of further heart attacks but of arterial disease in general, particularly intermittent claudication, foot ulcers and amputation. This is easier said than done; Mr Brown needs a lot of encouragement from the hospital staff but, most of all, the support of his family. His wife and children must understand why he needs to stop smoking as they are the ones best able to help him. Here are some general tips:

- Try to persuade other members of the family to stop; he can never hope to succeed if he is constantly tempted by seeing them smoke.
- See him frequently and praise him if he succeeds.
- Encourage him to keep himself occupied with a hobby or interest so that there is less time to think about smoking.

Longer-term rehabilitation

All too often, well-meaning medical advisers, family and friends are overprotective towards someone who has had a heart attack and frightened to let him get back to normal. Heart attacks can destroy self-confidence so a great deal of encouragement is needed during convalescence. Leaflets published by the British Heart Foundation are a good source of information.

Tell Mr Brown to increase his activity gradually from day to day provided this does not make him short of breath or cause chest pain. Urine tests before breakfast and 2 hours after his main meal 2 days a week will check that his diabetes is still under control, and a visit to clinic 4 weeks after discharge will give him an opportunity to discuss any problems that have cropped up. Like all diabetic patients of his age, he is at risk of foot ulcers and diabetic retinopathy, so education and regular examination will be an important part of his future care.

INSULIN-DEPENDENT DIABETES IN THE ELDERLY

Case History 8.2

Miss Hardy is an independent 81-year-old retired school teacher who has had diabetes for a year. Her general practitioner made the diagnosis when she complained that she was thirsty and losing weight. She was started on tablets and at first felt better and regained a few pounds in weight but remained thin. Recently she has started to lose weight again and become weak and forgetful. Her neighbours are worried because she has become incontinent. They suspect that she has cancer and are upset by the fact that she has apparently become senile.

The district nurse visits Miss Hardy, and tests her urine for diabetes. It is strongly positive for glucose and ketones.

Is ill-health in the elderly due to diabetes?

Of course, people with diabetes may have cancer or become demented like any other elderly person, but the first priority is to be sure that diabetes is not the cause of all their problems. Poor dia-

Table 8.3 Possible reasons for incontinence in an elderly person with diabetes

- Poor diabetic control
- Urinary tract infection
- Mechanical problems
  - Procidentia
  - Prostatism
  - Constipation
- Treatment with diuretics
- Dementia
- Neuropathic bladder due to diabetic autonomic neuropathy

betic control can cause tiredness, weakness, confusion and (by increasing the amount of urine passed) incontinence. If she had been able to test her urine herself, consistently positive results might have alerted Miss Hardy or her neighbours to the fact that her diabetes was out of control. However, many elderly people cannot do this because their eyesight is not good enough to read the results, they are too confused, they cannot handle the test strips or have not been taught slowly and patiently enough. In this case, weight loss is an important clue.

Most other causes of incontinence (Table 8.3) can be excluded by examining Miss Hardy, but will have to be reconsidered if it does not improve when her urine is free of glucose. By the same token, the only way to be sure that her weight loss and weakness are due to diabetes is to improve her control; other common causes of weight loss are summarised in Table 8.4.

Table 8.4 Possible reasons for weight loss in an elderly diabetic patient

- Poor diabetic control
- An overstrict diet
- Thyrotoxicosis
- Depression and social isolation
- Cancer (particularly pancreatic cancer), heart failure, tuberculosis or other serious underlying disease

Diagnosis of insulin-dependent diabetes in the elderly

The fact that Miss Hardy deteriorated steadily while treated with oral hypoglycaemics should have suggested that, despite being diagnosed diabetic aged 80, she has insulin-dependent diabetes just like little Mary Jenner (see Case History 3.1, page 42). Presence of ketones in the urine confirms this. Already thin, weak and losing weight, she needs insulin urgently and will slip into ketoacidosis and die without it. On insulin, she stands a good chance of regaining her former health and independence. But unlike David (see Case History 5.1, page 84), she is far too ill to stay at home and must start insulin in hospital.

Care of the elderly diabetic patient in hospital

No matter how frail and ill Miss Hardy may appear at first sight, do not forget that insulin might make a dramatic difference and allow her to regain her old independence. Skilled nursing care from the start could make the difference between success and failure. Before discussing insulin treatment and diet, here are some general points that are particularly important in someone with diabetes.

Beware pressure sores

Any elderly person who is thin and immobile is at risk of pressure sores; diabetes makes this even more likely by interfering with the nerve and blood supply to the skin of her back and feet. Regular turns, soft pads over the heels and under her bottom, sitting out of bed from the start and encouraging her to walk as soon as possible should help. A few hours of neglect at an early stage could cause ulcers over her heels which might take months to heal or lead to an amputation.

The indignity of incontinence

Quite apart from increasing the risk of pressure sores, incontinence is degrading. Skilled and sympathetic nursing care will keep up morale until the diabetes comes under control and incontinence (hopefully) improves.

Day clothes, routine and mobility as if at home

Nothing makes a person feel more like a 'patient' than a hospital nightgown. Even before Miss Hardy can walk independently, wearing her own clothes and having some of her own possessions on the bedside locker will help to preserve her own identity and dignity. She should sit out of bed from the start and be encouraged to walk as soon as her legs are strong enough. She may secretly fear that diabetes is going to make her an invalid for the rest of her life; the sooner she sees this is not true, the better. Even taking such modest exercise as walking to and from the toilet and kitchen burns up sugar and will lower her insulin requirements. It is impossible to judge how much insulin she will need at home unless she is encouraged to get into a similar routine in hospital. If she spends all her time sitting in a chair whilst her insulin doses are being adjusted in hospital, she may be hypoglycaemic within 24 h of getting home and immediately lose the self-confidence which has taken so long to build up.

Insulin treatment in the elderly

What sort and how much?

A single daily injection of medium-acting (isophane or lente) insulin often controls diabetes quite adequately in the elderly. It is best to start at a low dose (15–20 units, for example) and increase it at intervals of 3–4 days until symptoms are controlled and the patient starts to regain weight. Starting at a higher dose in the hope of controlling symptoms rapidly is a recipe for hypoglycaemic disaster later on! It is usually unnecessary to use more than one type of insulin but twice-daily injections may sometimes be needed to achieve acceptable control without hypoglycaemia.

Once Miss Hardy starts to regain weight (and, hopefully, her incontinence and confusion improve) her future management has to be thought out. This is a time when a nurse's enthusiasm in teaching the patient, coordinating services and supporting neighbours, friends and family is vital. The priorities for Miss Hardy's future care are summarised in Table 8.5 and discussed below.

Who should draw up and give the insulin?

Even people in their 80s may manage their own injections very well, although they are likely to take longer to learn and need

Table 8.5 Objectives for managing an elderly person with insulin-dependent diabetes

Treatment	An uncomplicated insulin regimen Simple, clear dietary advice
Control	Prevent hyperglycaemic coma (ketoacidosis) Prevent symptoms of hyperglycaemia Prevent hypoglycaemia
Education	Basic understanding of diabetes, hypoglycaemia, hyperglycaemia and the need for regular diet and insulin
Monitoring	Use well-being and weight as a guide to the success of therapy Occasional measurement of blood glucose or HbA_1 Monitoring of urine by patient, relative, friend or nurse if possible
Social support	Ensure adequate support from neighbours, family, social services
Screening	Check visual acuity, fundi and feet at least yearly for treatable diabetic complications

closer supervision in the early stages. Drawing up the insulin usually poses more of a problem than injecting it. Teaching should be kept simple and repeated as often as necessary; elderly people should be able to go through the whole procedure over and over again under supervision until they are either completely confident or obviously unable to manage. Mixing insulins is an unnecessary complication which should be avoided. If for any reason a mixture is required, one of the premixed formulations can be used (see Table 1.6). Poor eyesight may be an obstacle to drawing up insulin; various devices such as the 'click-count' and preset syringes, magnifying glasses which attach to ordinary syringes and free-standing magnifying glasses are available to overcome this problem (see page 121). Even patients who are unable to draw up their own insulin may still be able to inject it if syringes are prefilled and left in the fridge. These can be prepared several days in advance by a friend, relative or district nurse. Once-daily insulin is usually adequate and eases the burden if someone else has to give the injections. If twice-daily injections are necessary and the syringes have to be prefilled, much confusion can be avoided if both morning and evening doses are kept the same.

What should elderly diabetic patients eat?

Above all else, dietary advice must be simple and need be little different whether patients are treated with diet alone, tablets or insulin. It is unrealistic to expect the very elderly to stick to a carbohydrate exchange system. A simple diet sheet with sample menus may be helpful although there is a danger that they will never dare stray away from them. Even avoiding sugar may be very hard and is not absolutely essential. To prevent hypoglycaemia in patients on sulphonylureas or insulin, it is most important to stress the need to eat at least *three times a day*. Many old people prefer not to eat snacks between meals because they do not have big appetites, but a snack before bed is important to prevent nocturnal hypoglycaemia. If overweight, they should eat less at mealtimes and leave out snacks, and the dose of tablets or insulin should be reduced to avoid hypoglycaemia. Exactly what they eat is less important and may be determined by what is available. Many prefer to take their main meal at lunchtime; there is no need for this to be changed. Elderly people often follow the advice they are given to the letter. Unless they are told that eating the 'forbidden foods' (cakes, chocolates and puddings) occasionally will do them no harm, they may be deprived of one of their main pleasures in life and condemned to a monotonous diet. Similarly, if all that is available is a sugary pudding, it is better to have this and risk transient hyperglycaemia than to miss it out and go hypo.

Monitoring diabetes in the elderly

Asking about the symptoms of hyperglycaemia is not always helpful because old people may not be thirsty even when their diabetes is wildly out of control. It is important to ask if they pass urine at night—this may suggest poor control. Body weight is a good guide to health in the elderly which is often forgotten; it is quite simple to weigh someone once a week. Uncontrolled diabetes for more than 2 or 3 days will always cause them to lose weight, although the other causes of weight loss (see Table 8.4) must also be borne in mind. If Miss Hardy *gained* weight excessively, this would indicate that she was eating too much. Urine testing is a useful warning of poor control; Miss Hardy would probably never have become so ill in the first place if her urine had been checked from time to time. If she cannot see well enough to do her own tests, arrangements can be made for a nurse to call weekly to see how she is and test her urine. An occasional blood test for glucose or HbA_1 will be useful but is not essential.

Hypoglycaemia in the elderly

Keeping a watch out for hypoglycaemia is most important since it may be frightening and dangerous. It can usually be avoided by not aiming for overtight control. If it does occur, the elderly may not complain of the typical symptoms of sweating, lightheadedness and shakiness before meals; confusion, falls or excessive weight gain may be the only clues. A blood sugar may not be diagnostic unless by chance it is actually taken during hypoglycaemia. HbA_1 (see page 26) may be more helpful; a level which is well within the normal range may indicate that good control has been achieved at the expense of hypoglycaemia. It may be necessary to cut down the insulin dose for a trial period to see if matters improve.

Social supports for the elderly diabetic patient

Involving a social worker soon after the patient is admitted to hospital will help to identify her particular needs and ensure that they can be met when she is discharged. As with other elderly people, regular visitors will help the elderly diabetic to cope at home and should be encouraged. Miss Hardy's home help and family probably know nothing about diabetes. The diabetes liaison sister could usefully prepare for her discharge by arranging to meet them at her home. The most useful things they can do is to check that she is taking her injections and meals regularly and keep a watch on her general state of health. Although depending on someone else to draw up insulin creates demands, it does ensure that she is visited each day. Most important of all, they need to have the telephone number of the diabetes ward or a nurse who can give advice when needed.

Screening for diabetic complications in the elderly

Once the hurdle of managing insulin treatment at home has been overcome, Miss Hardy needs to be examined periodically for early signs of treatable complications. Old people may not complain of poor eyesight, even when they are nearly blind, but detecting retinopathy and cataracts early may save their eyesight (see pages 116–18). Similarly, foot ulcers may be painless due to neuropathy and can rapidly lead to gangrene and amputation if not spotted in time (see pages 151–9). A nurse or doctor should be contacted at the first sign of an ulcer or blister; meticulous care of ulcers, chiropody and suitable footwear will help avoid disasters.

Should the patient attend a hospital clinic?

Elderly people with diabetes often have to attend several hospital clinics, each looking after different problems—for example, an ophthalmic clinic, a general medical or diabetic clinic and a chiropodist. It is easy to forget that these entail long, uncomfortable ambulance rides, a lot of hanging about and much expense for the health service. Clinic attendances should be kept to the minimum and coordinated so that they take place on the same day if at all possible. Doctors are often unaware of these sort of problems so a district nurse can do a lot of good by pointing them out. If the patient does not need hospital care, regular visits from her general practitioner, chiropody and yearly visits to the optician can provide all that a clinic has to offer. If a foot ulcer or other problem develops, she can be seen promptly in clinic.

STROKE IN THE ELDERLY DIABETIC

Case History 8.3

Clara Sutton, a 70-year-old widow, has been diabetic for 10 years. Since the death of her husband, she has become increasingly confused and forgetful and her family are worried that she is not safe to live alone. One morning her son calls in and finds her lying on the kitchen floor. He calls an ambulance and she is taken to casualty. She is not moving her right arm or leg. Her bottles of tablets, including glibenclamide, are given to the casualty sister.

Table 8.6 Causes of collapse or confusion in an elderly diabetic patient

- Hypoglycaemia
- Severe hyperglycaemia (ketoacidosis)
- Stroke
- Epileptic fit
- Heart attack
- Urinary infection, chest infection or septicaemia
- Drug side-effect or overdose
- Hypothyroidism
- Hypothermia
- Dementia
- Excess alcohol

'Collapse' in an elderly diabetic patient

There are many causes, summarised in Table 8.6. The first to be considered in Mrs Sutton's case is hypoglycaemia. Like other sulphonylureas (particularly chlorpropamide), glibenclamide can cause profound and prolonged hypoglycaemia. This may mimic a stroke, even to the extent of causing weakness down one side of the body although the weakness usually recovers almost immediately when treated. Hypoglycaemia can be excluded by a blood test, but the other problems listed in Table 8.6 require a detailed history, physical examination and investigations. Typically, Mrs Sutton will be admitted to an elderly persons' ward.

Care of a diabetic patient after a stroke

How should she be monitored and treated?

Glibenclamide is a potent drug which acts for over 24 h. Mrs Sutton can take little by mouth as a result of her stroke. Assuming she took her normal pill earlier in the day, she might easily become hypoglycaemic after admission, even if her blood glucose was slightly high in casualty. Urine tests cannot detect hypoglycaemia, so her blood glucose needs to be checked at the bedside every 4 h for the first 24 h. Even when the risk of hypoglycaemia has passed, it would be reasonable to stop glibenclamide temporarily to see if tablets are still needed.

Once past the acute phase, checking the urine four times a day for glucose should be perfectly adequate; provided the patient has less than 1% glycosuria, her diabetes is not seriously out of control. If the tests become strongly positive, her blood glucose should be checked and the urine tested for ketones. An old person who is unable to eat may well have a trace of ketones in the urine (*starvation ketones*). This is not a sign of uncontrolled diabetes if there is no glucose in the urine and the blood glucose is 13 mmol/l or below. If her diabetes slips out of control (urine glucose consistently 1% or higher, blood glucose above 13 mmol/l with or without ketones in the urine), twice-daily insulin would be the best way of controlling it until she is over the acute phase of her stroke and can swallow tablets. Patients on insulin before admission should be monitored in exactly the same way and insulin continued, but the dose would probably need to be reduced to prevent hypoglycaemia.

Diet

Patients with strokes often have difficulty swallowing so the first priority is to encourage fluids to prevent dehydration. At first Mrs Sutton will only be able to manage sloppy foods like porridge, soup, puddings and icecream. Once she can manage a more normal diet it is sensible to find foods which interest her rather than to restrict what she eats because she is diabetic.

Other important points

General nursing care of the elderly diabetic patient in hospital has already been discussed. The importance of preventing pressure sores cannot be overemphasised. With her long history of confusion and an acute stroke, a patient like Mrs Sutton will need residential care. Now the task is to advise the staff of the nursing home how to look after her, best achieved by a visit from the diabetes liaison nurse.

Telling the staff of an old peoples' home about diabetes

Remember first that many lay people are afraid of diabetes. They immediately think of insulin injections, have vaguely heard of hypoglycaemia and assume that looking after someone with diabetes will be a fearsome responsibility. In fact, the objectives are quite straightforward (see Table 8.5): to keep Mrs Sutton free of diabetic symptoms; to prevent hyperglycaemic coma; and to prevent her from losing or putting on too much weight. The nurse's task is to reassure the staff of the home that Mrs Sutton does not need tablets or insulin and explain the aims of her diet to them.

What should she eat?

This depends on the facilities available in the home. The principles have already been discussed (see page 178). If the home can easily provide a diet with little sugar and plenty of high fibre foods, so much the better. In this case, the staff might appreciate the opportunity to discuss her diet with a dietitian. However, all too often an attempt to provide a diabetic diet means scanty portions, unappetising foods, little variety and a punitive attitude from the staff if Mrs Sutton ever eats sugar. There is no real need to prepare special foods; the diabetic patient can eat the same as the other residents, but the secret of success is to take everything in moderation, particularly sweet foods like cakes. However, it must be emphasised that a piece of cake at Christmas time and on her birthday will do no harm! Like children, the elderly feel cheated if they are deprived of treats.

Monitoring diabetes and seeking advice

The staff need to weigh Mrs Sutton once a month and keep a watch on her general well-being. It would be helpful if they could learn to do urine tests, though this is not essential; a urine test before breakfast several days a week should suffice. Of course, occasional positive urine tests do not matter, but consistently positive tests before breakfast together with hyperglycaemic symptoms and weight loss are a warning sign of uncontrolled diabetes and help should be sought at once. Giving nursing home staff the telephone number of the hospital ward or diabetes unit will give them confidence in looking after the patient. The general practitioner responsible for the nursing home may also be called to advise; much confusion can be avoided if the plan for Mrs Sutton's management is discussed with him when she is discharged from hospital.

Further reading

Keen H., Jarrett R. J. (eds) (1982) *Diabetic Complications*, 2nd edn. London: Edward Arnold. Diabetes and heart disease.

Tattersall R. B. (1984) Diabetes in the elderly. *Diabetologia*; **27**: 167–173.

Appendix 1

One dose injection

The step-by-step routine for measuring your insulin from one bottle

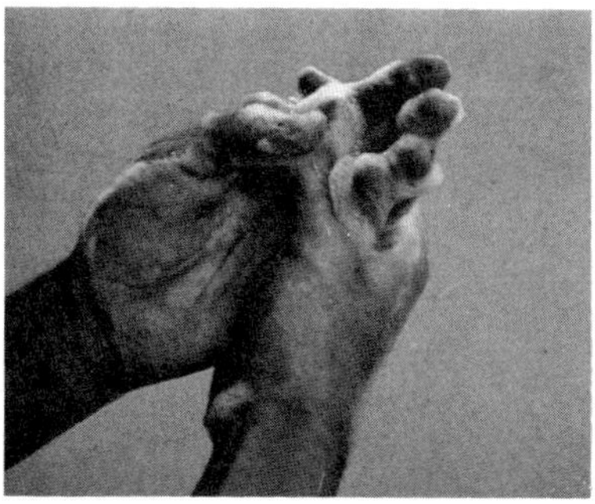

1. Wash your hands and dry them

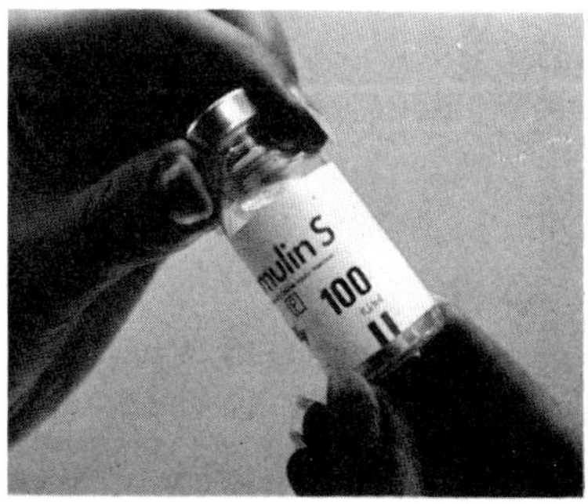

2. Check the label on the insulin bottle for any special instructions

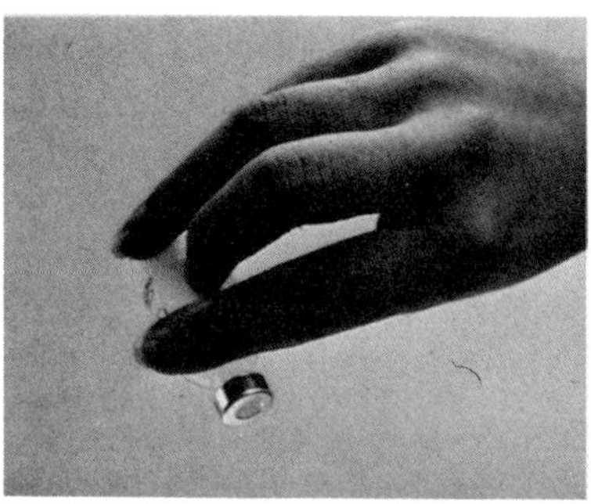

3. Clean the rubber cap of the bottle with cottonwool and industrial spirit or with a single-use alcohol swab

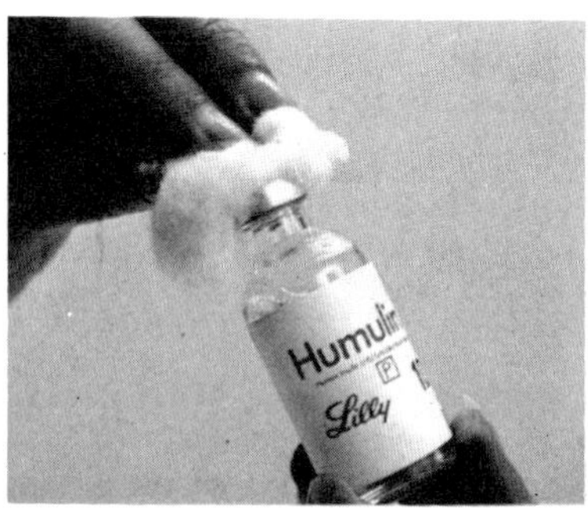

4. Gently tip the bottle to and fro to make sure that the insulin is properly mixed. This is especially important when using cloudy insulin

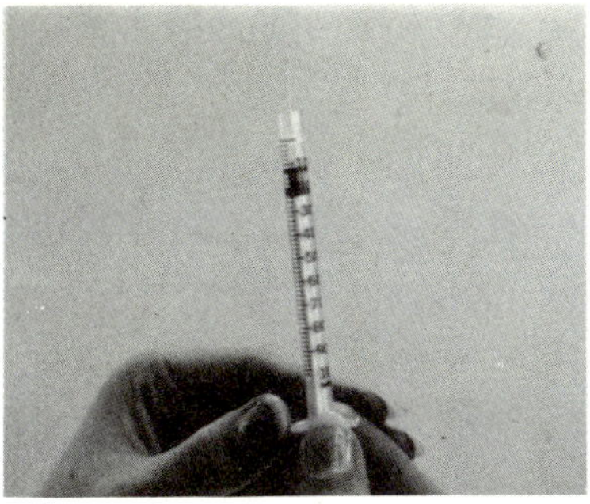

5. Pull back the plunger of the syringe to measure approximately the same amount of air as the amount of insulin you use

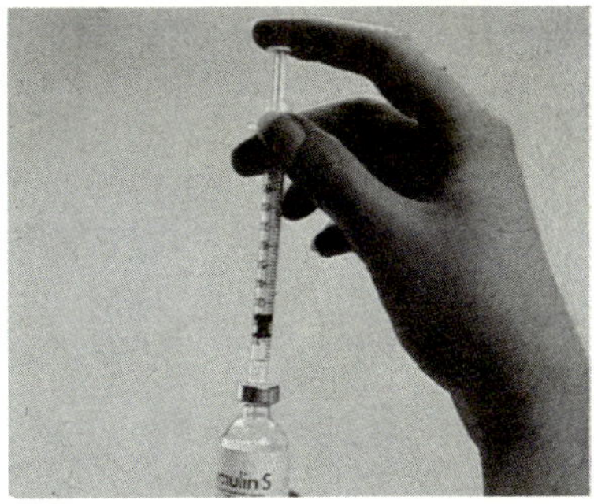

6. Insert the needle straight through the rubber cap of the insulin bottle and inject the air into the bottle

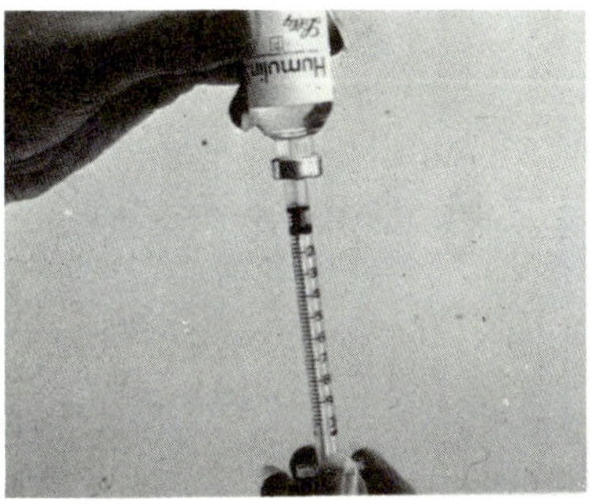

7. Now turn the bottle upside down. Make certain that the point of the needle inside the bottle is well beneath the surface level of the insulin

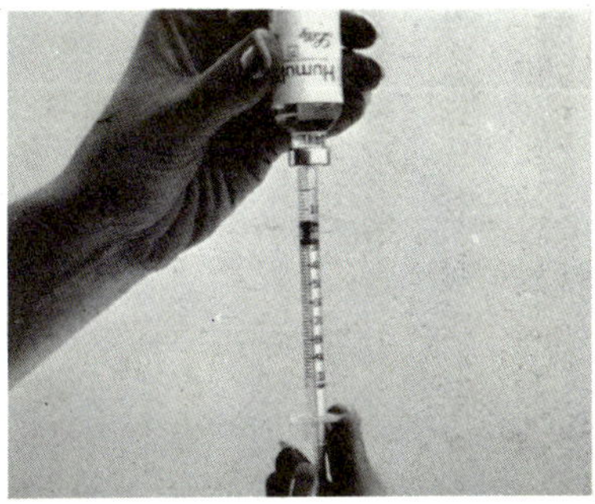

8. Continue holding the bottle and syringe upright with the point upwards and pull back the plunger until you have measured slightly more than your correct dose of insulin

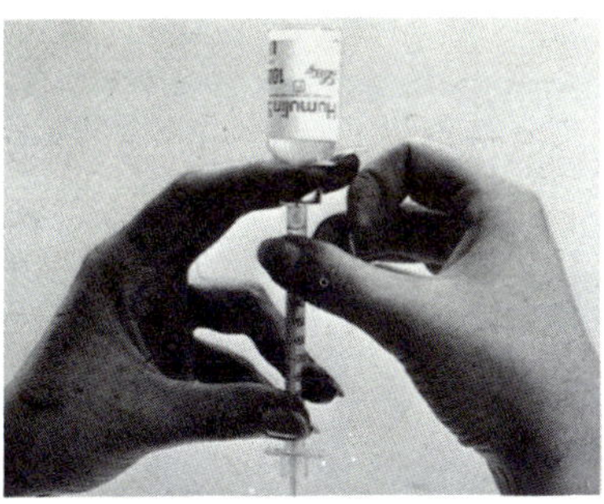

9. If any air bubbles have entered the syringe, tap the syringe barrel fairly gently with your finger and this will usually release them so that they rise to the tip of the syringe
NOTE: If the air bubbles persist, expel all of the insulin back into the bottle and start again

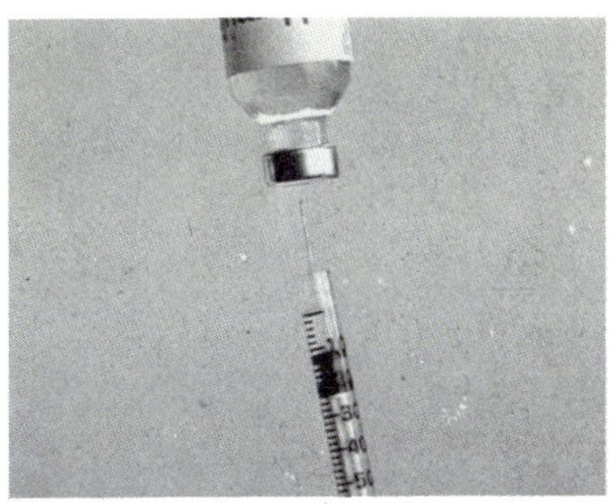

10. Press the plunger slightly to expel the bubbles back into the bottle. Adjust the plunger to measure your exact insulin dose and take the needle out of the bottle

Appendix 2

Mixed dose injection

If you use two types of insulin for a mixed dose then this is the way to do it

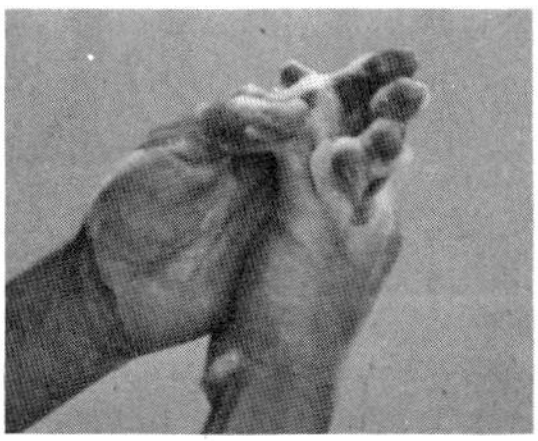

1. Wash your hands and dry them

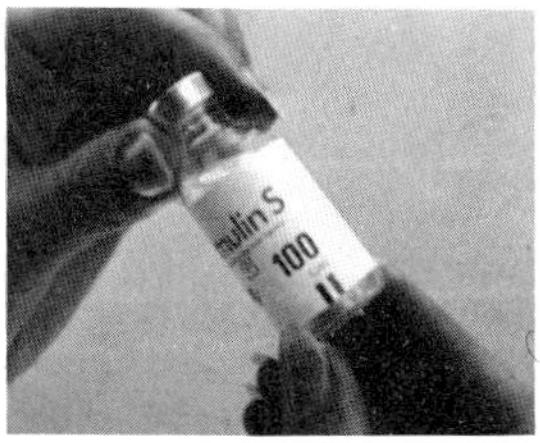

2. Check the labels on the insulin bottles for any special instructions

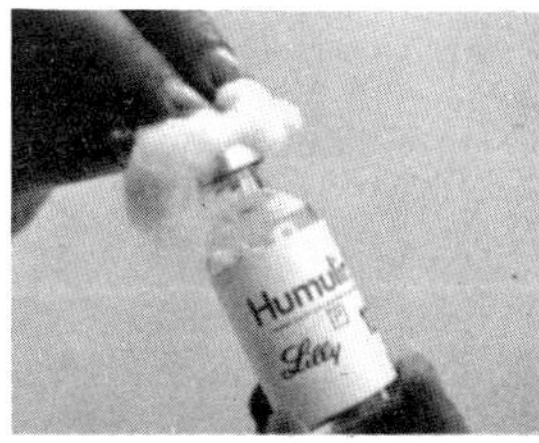

3. Clean the rubber caps of the bottle with cottonwool and industrial spirit or with a single-use alcohol swab

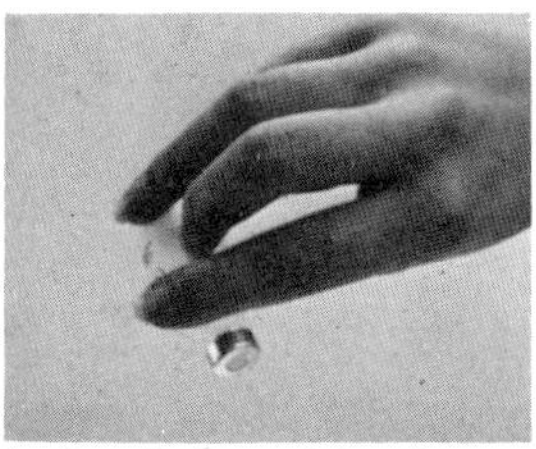

4. Gently tip each bottle to and fro to make sure that the insulin is properly mixed; this is especially important for the cloudy insulins

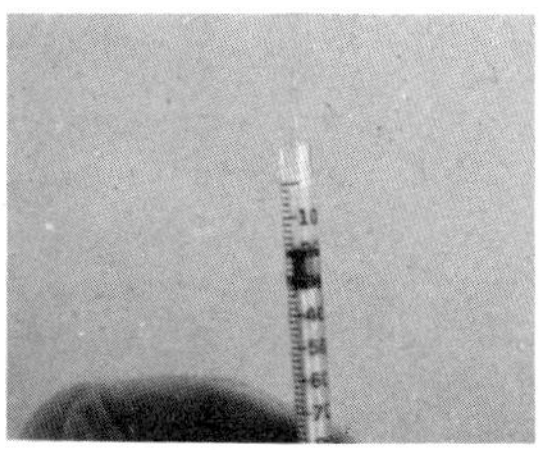

5. Pull back the plunger of the syringe to measure approximately the same amount of air as the amount of *cloudy* insulin that you use

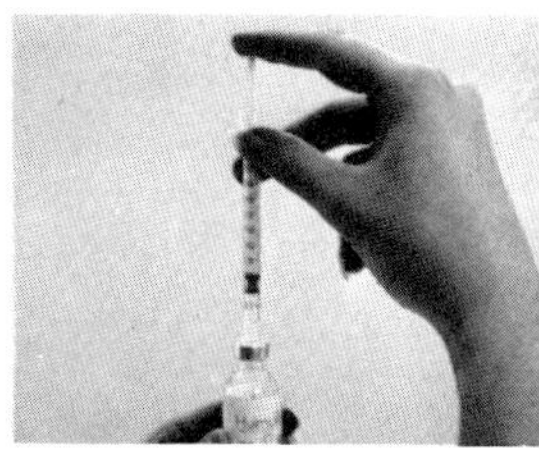

6. Insert the needle straight though the rubber cap of the *cloudy* insulin bottle and inject the air into the bottle

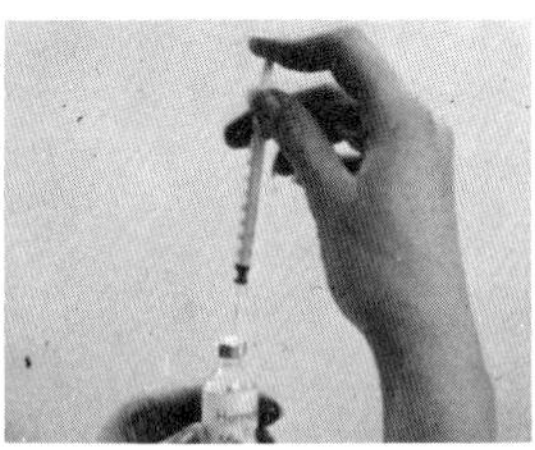

6a. Keep the plunger fully pressed down and *remove the needle from the bottle*

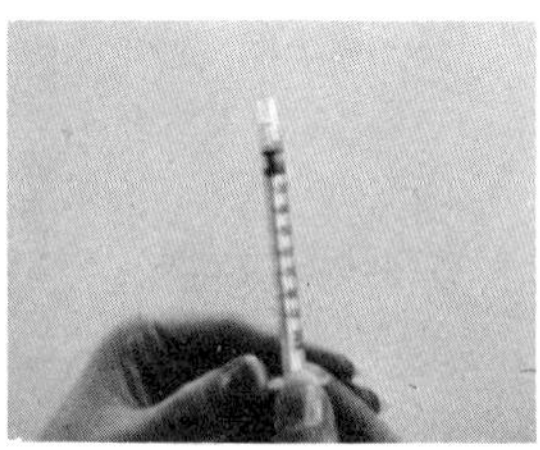

7. Pull back the plunger of the syringe to measure approximately the same amount of air as the amount of *clear* insulin that you use

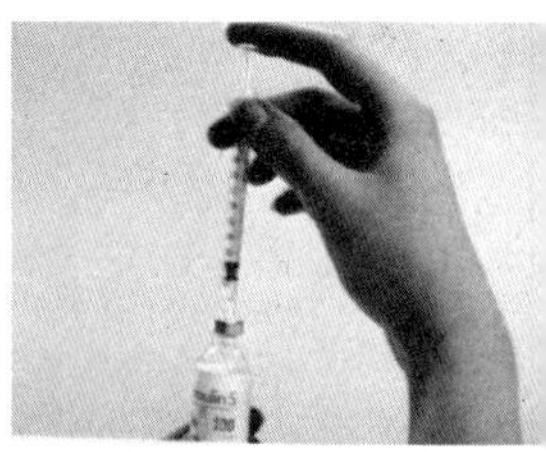

8. Insert the needle straight through the rubber cap of the *clear* insulin bottle and inject the air into the bottle

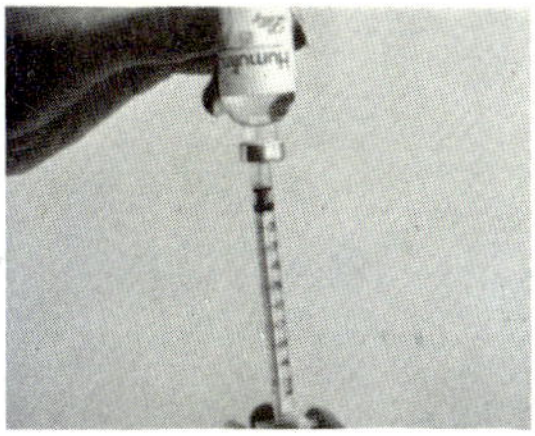

9. Now turn the bottle upside down; make certain that the point of the needle inside the bottle is well beneath the surface level of the insulin

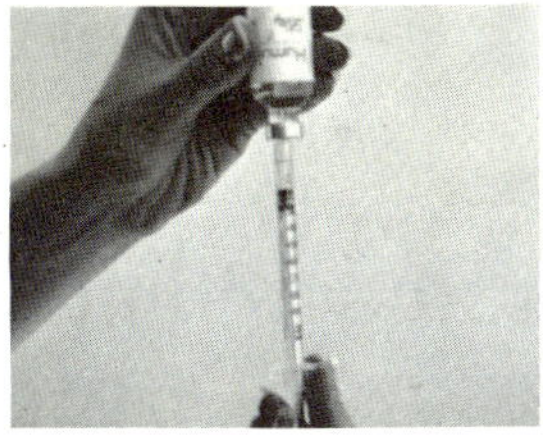

10. Continue holding the bottle and syringe upright with the point upwards and pull back the plunger until you have measured slightly more than your correct dose of *clear* insulin

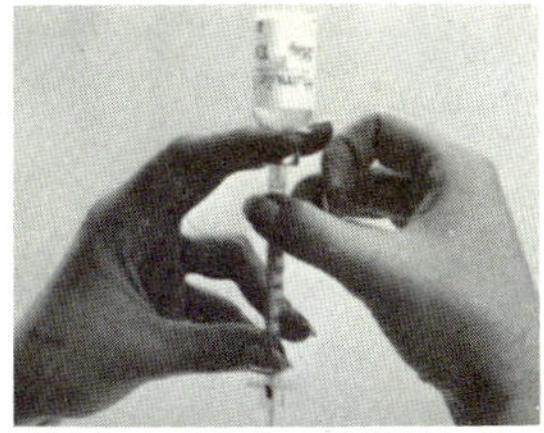

11. If any air bubbles have entered the syringe, tap the syringe barrel fairly gently with your finger and this will usually release them so that they rise to the tip of the syringe.
NOTE: If any air bubbles persist, expel all of the *clear* insulin back into the bottle and start again

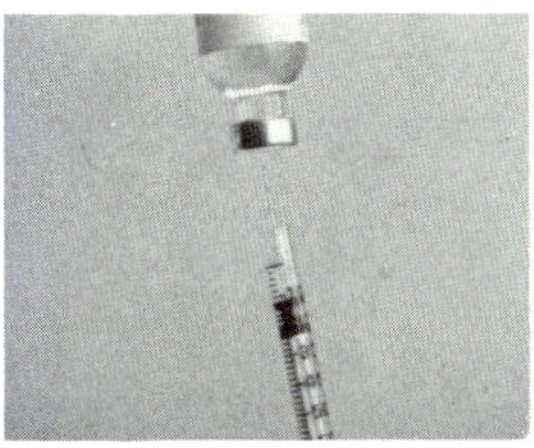

12. Press the plunger slightly to expel the bubbles back into the bottle. Adjust the plunger to measure your exact dose of *clear* insulin. Withdraw the needle from the bottle

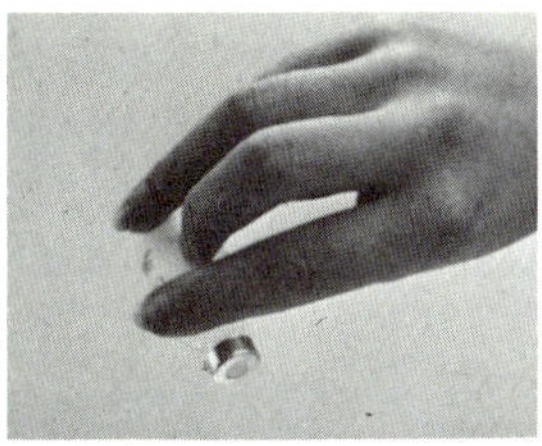

13. Once again, gently tip the *cloudy* insulin bottle to and fro to make sure that the insulin is properly mixed

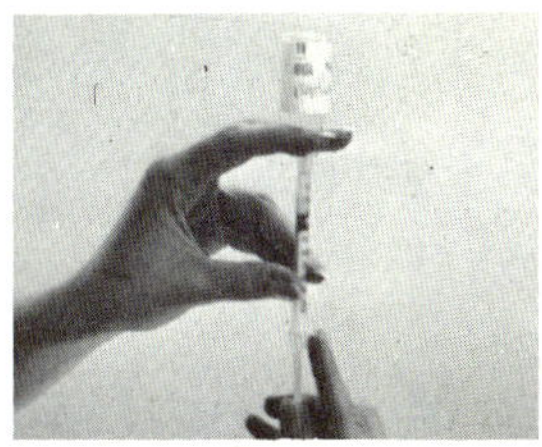

14. Now reinsert the needle into the upturned bottle of *cloudy* insulin. Make certain that the point of the needle inside the bottle is well beneath the surface level of the insulin. Carefully pull back the plunger until you have measured your *exact* dose of *cloudy* insulin.

14a

VERY IMPORTANT

If you accidentally measure too much *cloudy* insulin *DO NOT* press the plunger and return the excess amount into the bottle because some *clear* insulin will also be injected into the *cloudy* insulin bottle. Just remove the needle from the bottle, press the plunger to the bottom and discharge all of the insulin from the syringe into the sink. Then start again from 5

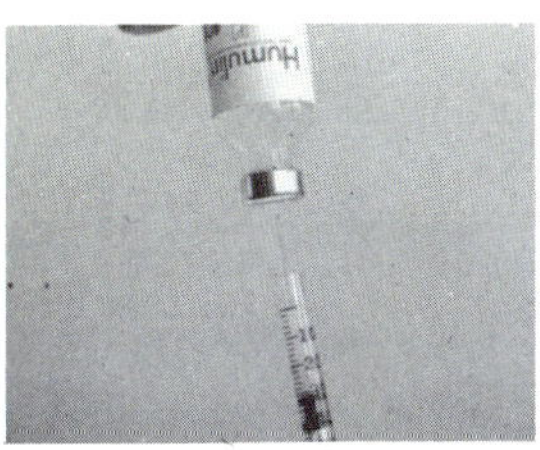

15. Withdraw the needle from the *cloudy* bottle

15a.

VERY IMPORTANT

ALWAYS measure your two insulins in the same order every day

Appendix 3

How to inject

METHOD ONE

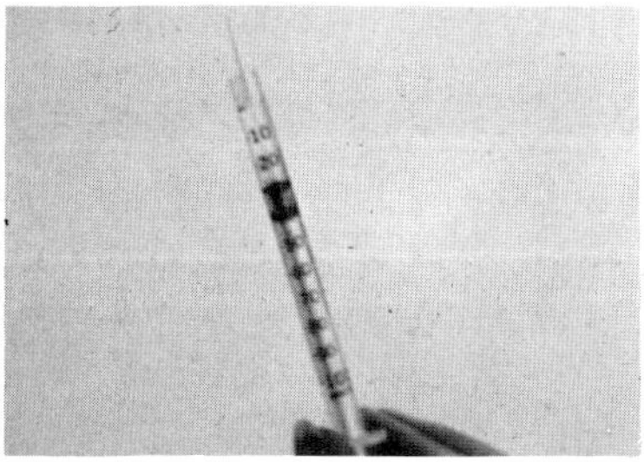

1. Make absolutely certain once again that you have measured your insulin dose to the correct mark on the syringe

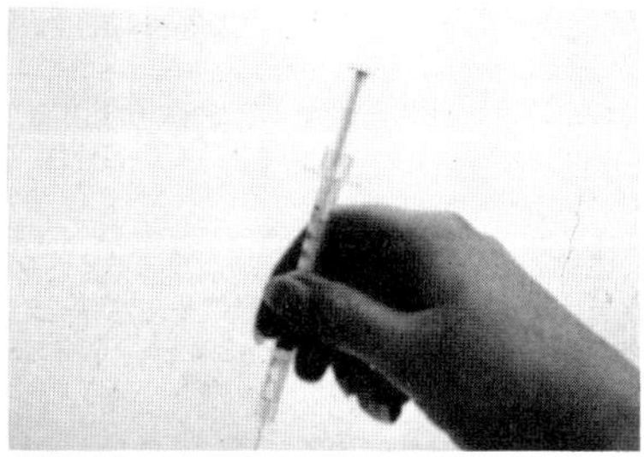

2. Taking care not to touch the sterile needle, hold the syringe firmly near the top, as if you were going to write with it like a pencil

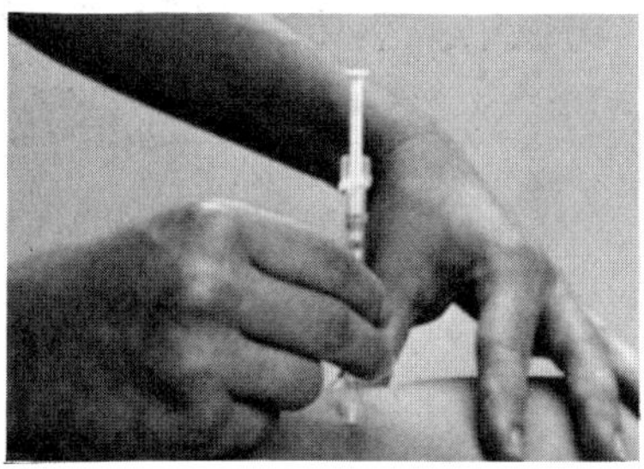

3. Now, using the thumb and forefinger of the other hand, stretch flat an area of clean skin and quickly push the needle straight in as far as it will go

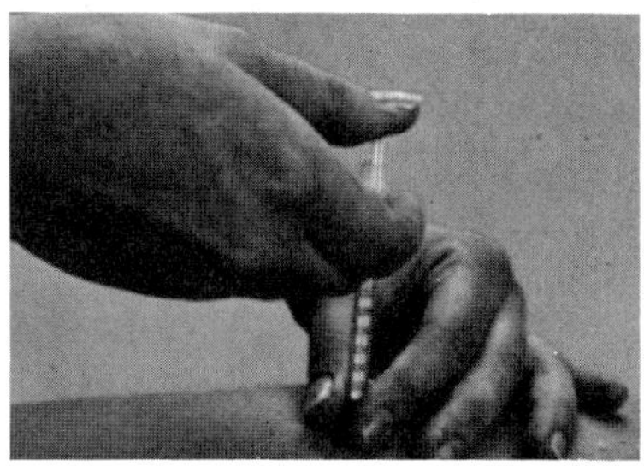

4. Hold the syringe barrel comfortably in place with one hand so that your other hand is free to press the plunger. With your thumb on top of the plunger, quickly and smoothly inject all of the insulin in the syringe

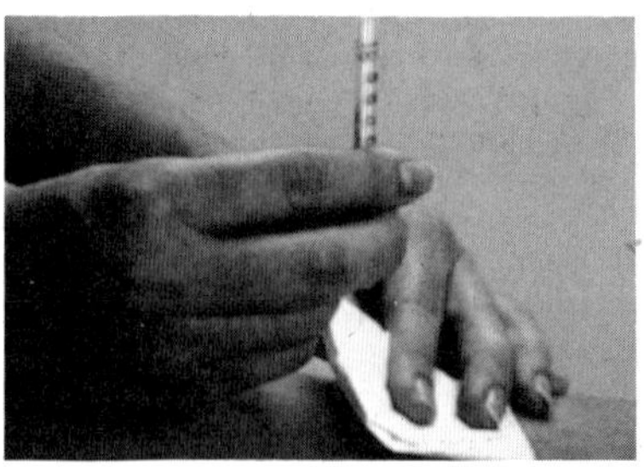

5. Withdraw the needle and quickly place a clean piece of tissue or cottonwool over the injection site. Hold it in place with firm pressure for just a few seconds. Your injection is completed

METHOD TWO

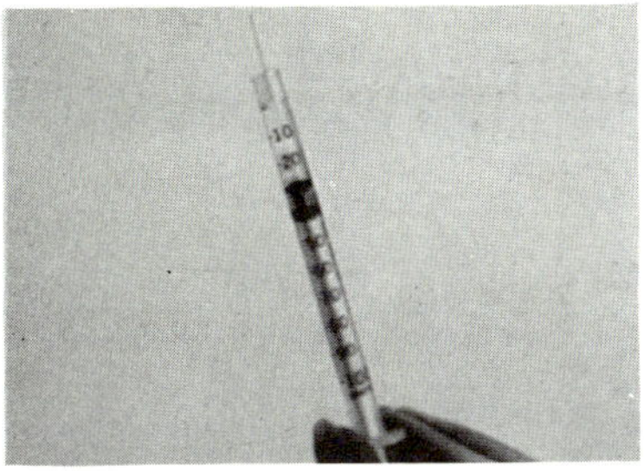

1. Make absolutely certain once again that you have measured your insulin dose to the correct mark on the syringe

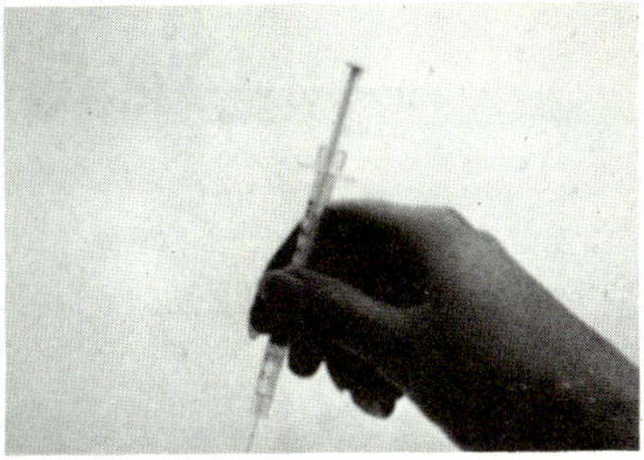

2. Taking care not to touch the sterile needle, hold the syringe firmly near the top, as if you were going to write with it like a pencil

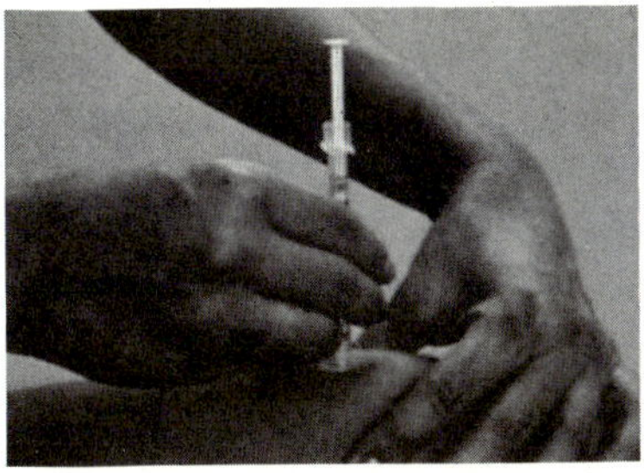

3. Now, using the other hand, pinch up a mound of clean skin and quickly push the needle straight into the mound as far as it will go. (Some people prefer to insert the needle at a slight angle—almost vertical but not quite)

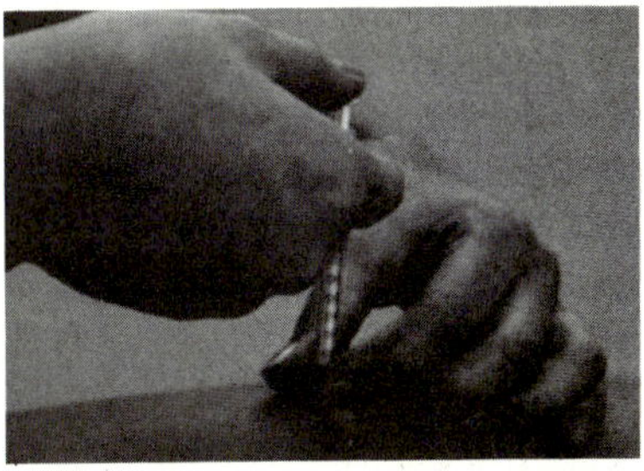

4. Release the mound of skin. Hold the syringe barrel comfortably in place with one hand so that your other hand is free to press the plunger. With your thumb on top of the plunger, quickly and smoothly inject all of the insulin in the syringe

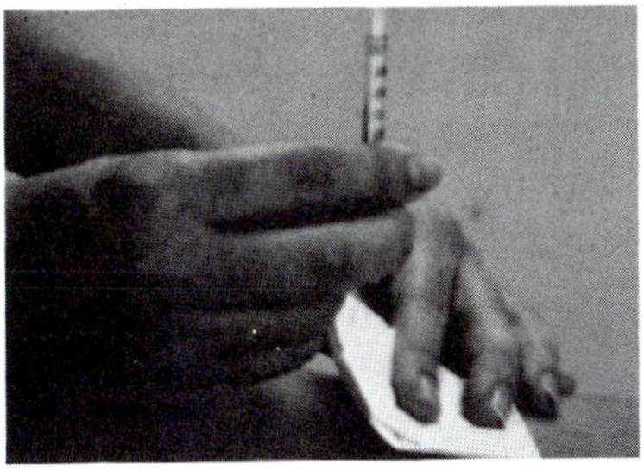

5. Withdraw the needle and quickly place a clean piece of tissue or cottonwool over the injection site. Hold it in place with firm pressure for just a few seconds. Your injection is completed

IMPORTANT Your doctor or the nursing staff at your hospital are the final authorities regarding precisely how you should inject and the site of injection. Follow their advice carefully. The above two methods of injection are those that many people consider to be the easiest and the best

Appendix 4

Urine glucose test

Instructions for use

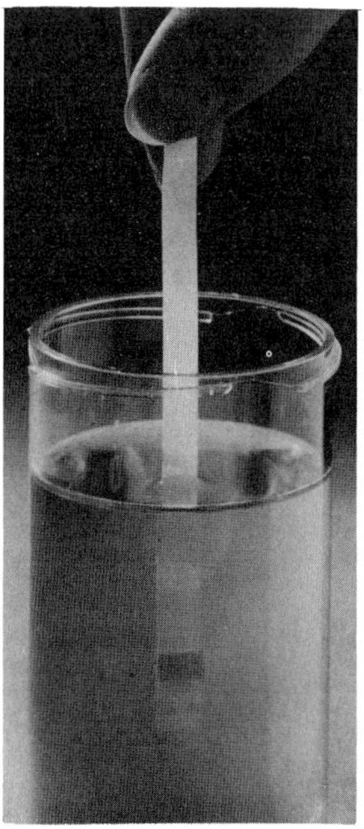

1. Collect a urine specimen in a clean container. Briefly dip the test strip into the urine

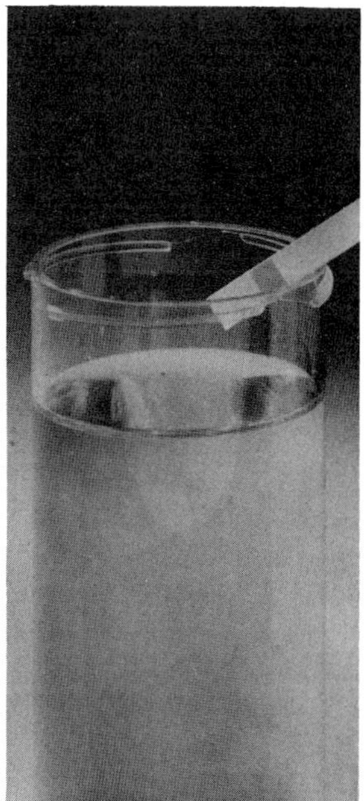

2. Withdraw and wipe edge along the rim of the container in order to remove excess urine

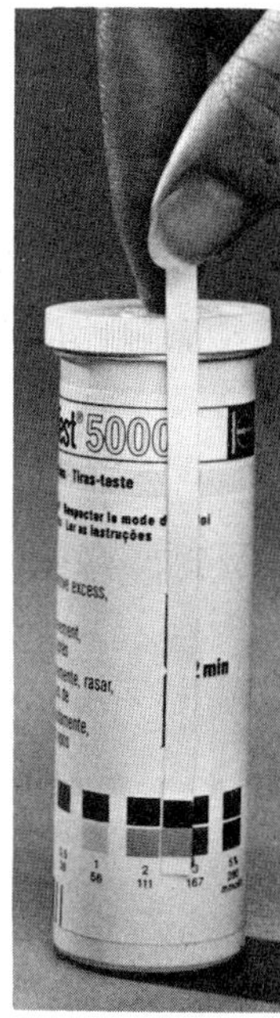

3. After 2 min compare the test areas with the colour scale on the label*

Alternative method

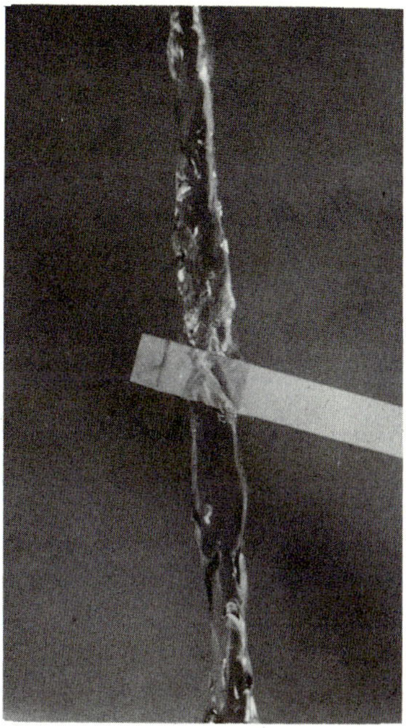

1. Briefly wet the test area by placing directly in the URINE STREAM. Shake off excess urine

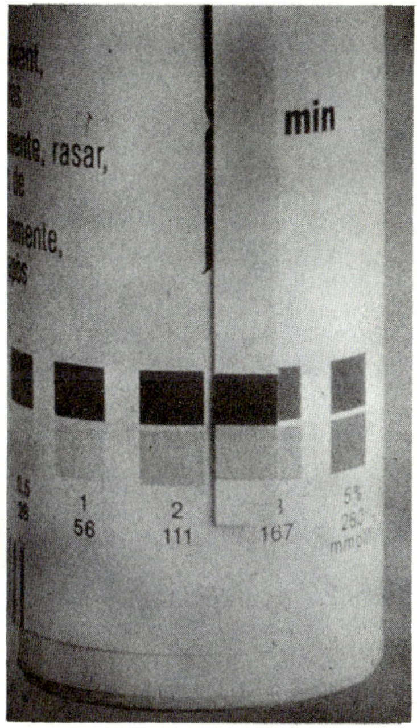

2. After 2 min compare the test areas with the colour scale*

* If no colour has developed after 1 min the result is negative.

Appendix 5

How to do a fingerprick blood test

How to check your blood glucose level using the BM-Test-Glycemie 1-44 test strip

Following these instructions will enable you to obtain a dependable result using BM-Test-Glycemie 1-44

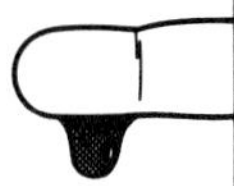

1. Obtain a good sized drop of blood – large enough to cover both test zones completely

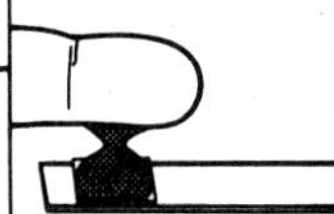

2. Place test strip on a flat clean surface. Apply sample – don't let skin touch test zones. Start timing

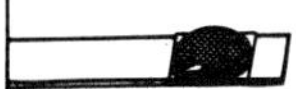

3. Leave blood on test zone for one minute. (Never spread or smear the blood

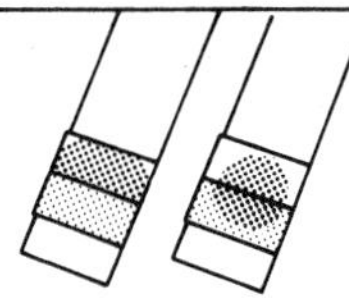

Good technique
1. Ideal – a good sized drop of blood has covered both test areas.
2. The smallest coverage that will give a definite result.

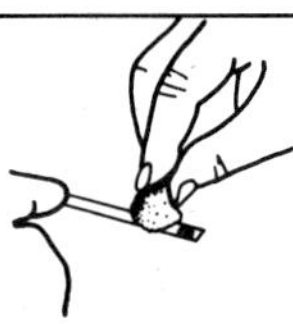

4. Hold test strip firmly against flat surface. Wipe with clean ball of cotton wool – repeat twice with clean area of wool. Leave test strip for one more minute

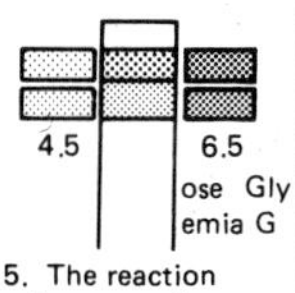

5. The reaction colours remain stable giving you ample time to read or recheck your results. Compare test zone with colour blocks on label of vial. Record your result

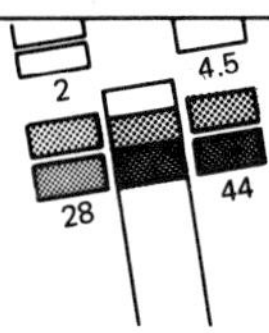

6. If your reading at 2 min is above 17 mmol/l, the reaction is not complete. Leave for a further minute and read again

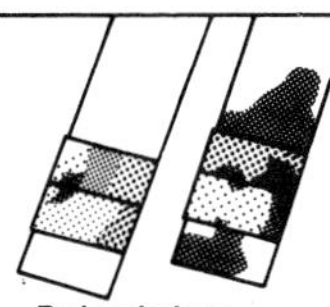

Bad technique
3. Results are unreliable – smearing has produced uneven colours.
4. Reading is impossible – blood stains on strip are due to inadequate wiping.

Reading results (interpretation)
IMPORTANT: Use the colour chart on the test strip vial itself when reading the reacted strip

When reading values below 9 mmol/l give priority to the block which matches the colour on the lower light blue test zone

When reading values above 9 mmol/l give priority to the block which matches the colour on the upper sage/deep green test zone

Appendix 6

Injecting glucagon

ADMINISTRATION GUIDE

Glucagon has the opposite effect to insulin. If a diabetic has a severe hypo and particularly if they become unconscious glucagon may be injected under the skin.

When the diabetic becomes conscious, carbohydrate such as milk must be given to prevent the hypo recurring.

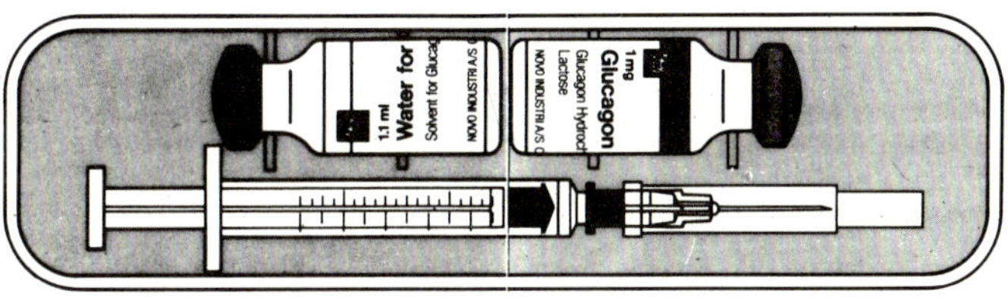

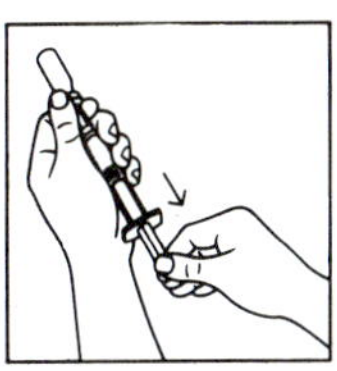

Use the disposable syringe provided to draw up the water for injections

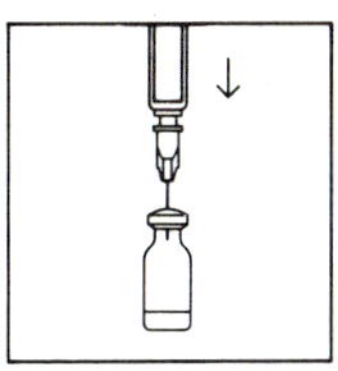

Inject the water for injections into the vial containing freeze-dried glucagon

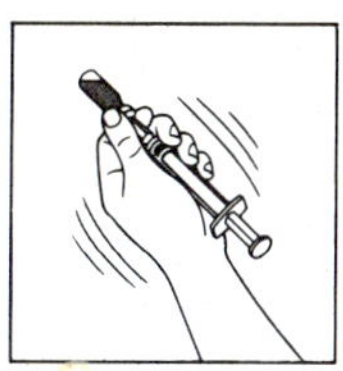

Without withdrawing the syringe, shake the vial until the contents are completely dissolved

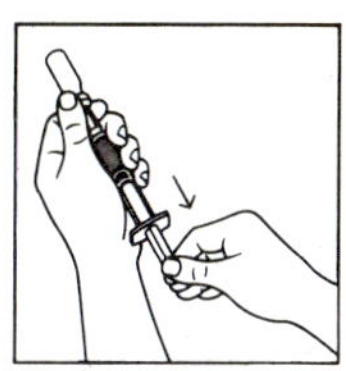

Draw up the solution into the syringe and inject it under the skin of the outer thigh or upper arm (subcutaneously). When the patient responds administer oral carbohydrate (such as Dextrosol, sweet biscuits or a sweet drink) to prevent a further hypo

Index